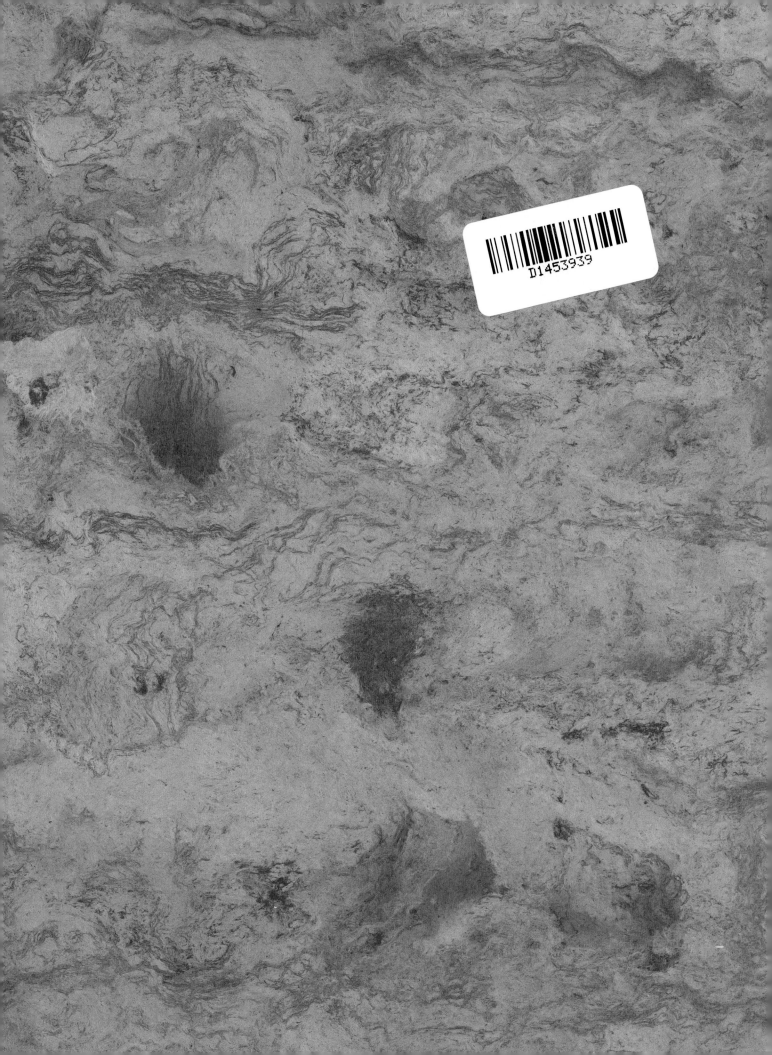

An Illustrated History of Hairstyles
1830-1930
Marian I. Doyle

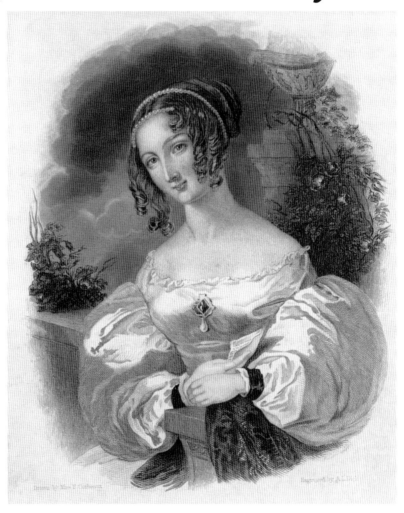

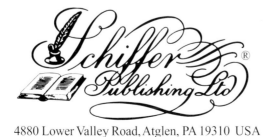

4880 Lower Valley Road, Atglen, PA 19310 USA

Dedication

I would like to dedicate this book to my husband, Phillip Doyle, whose patient help and understanding made it all possible.

Library of Congress Cataloging-in-Publication Data

Doyle, Marian I.
  An illustrated history of hairstyles 1830-1930 / by
Marian I. Doyle.
     p. cm.
  ISBN 0-7643-1734-2 (Hardcover)
1. Hairstyles--United States--History. 2. Hairstyles--History--
19th century. I. Title.
GT2295.U5D69 2003
391.5--dc21

2002156069

Designed by Mark David Bowyer
Type set in Zapf Calligraphy BT/Humanst521 BT

ISBN: 0-7643-1734-2
Printed in China

Published by Schiffer Publishing Ltd.
4880 Lower Valley Road
Atglen, PA 19310
Phone: (610) 593-1777; Fax: (610) 593-2002
E-mail: Info@schifferbooks.com
Please visit our web site catalog at www.schifferbooks.com
We are always looking for people to write books on new and related subjects. If you have an idea for a book, please contact us at the above address.

This book may be purchased from the publisher.
Include $3.95 for shipping.
Please try your bookstore first.
You may write for a free catalog.

In Europe, Schiffer books are distributed by
Bushwood Books
6 Marksbury Avenue
Kew Gardens
Surrey TW9 4JF England
Phone: 44 (0) 20 8392 8585
Fax: 44 (0) 20 8392 9876
E-mail: Bushwd@aol.com
Free postage in the UK. Europe: air mail at cost.

Contents

Preface

An Illustrated History of Hairstyles is a compilation of hair fashion from the past. It is visual history intended as a guide for those who stage reenactments or theatrical productions as well as for anyone puzzling over the age of a vintage picture. Extensive research alongside comparisons to period sources was employed to chronologically arrange these images as accurately as possible.

Not many old photographs come complete with names and dates, making attribution a problem. The first clues to age are found in the photograph itself—size, format, backing and photographer's imprint. Posing style, backdrop and furniture tell us more, though some studios were more advanced and profitable than others.

Clothing, jewelry, accessories and, of course, the hairstyles all help narrow the probable time of the sitting; but even here there are no certainties. A dress bodice that matches exactly the example on an 1867 fashion page may have been years old at the time the photographer snapped the picture. Some people simply lacked the means to stay perfectly in vogue while others held onto a favorite mode far beyond its time. The elderly in particular were loath to change.

Another confusing factor is the tendency of some fashions to repeat themselves at intervals. This is especially true of men's clothing where the width of a lapel or height of a collar may be the only distinguishing feature of a time period. Further, even the most hard and fast fashion rules of any given era could be violated by the individualist or the person with no eye for style. One final complication arises when families have had older photographs reproduced—a gentleman of the early 1870s might be found on card stock of the 1890s.

Despite these complexities and vagaries, a fascinating timeline of hair fashion emerges when representative images of the young, the old, the poor, and the wealthy are presented in progression. *An Illustrated History of Hairstyles* divides portrait examples and period illustrations into sections of women, men, children, and the aging, along with two additional chapters of hairdressing information. Where exact dates are known, they are given. Where unknown, the probable date of the photograph within a two to three year period is generally suggested.

The gathering together of material for this book was a project with frequent surprises. Eccentric hairstyles were found in every era, providing much humor but little useful data, and with a few exceptions they have been excluded. It is hoped that what remains is an informative, entertaining and easy to use guide to the way mainstream Americans once wore their hair.

Chapter One
A Small Deception

To understand American hairstyles of the past it is first necessary to recognize the role that supplemental hair played in their arrangement. Nearly every woman of the Victorian era owned at least one false hairpiece, whether an elaborately pre-styled chignon or a fringe of curls on a comb. It was a small deception with which they were comfortable, unapologetically buying falls, switches, braids and frizettes from shops and mail order houses across the country.

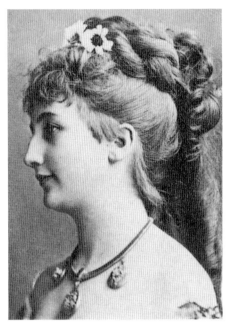

Ornate Victorian styles required more hair than any single head could produce.

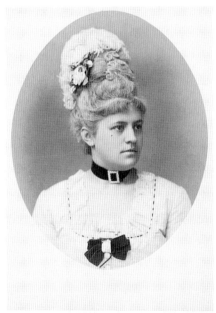

Towering 18th century coiffures demanded enormous amounts of padding and false hair, as in this theatrical creation of 1877.

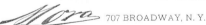

707 BROADWAY, N.Y.

Ridiculously high, ornate coiffures were historically popularized by Madame Pompadour and Marie Antoinette, whose hairdresser boasted of using fourteen yards of lace and gauze to build one of his elaborate "towers." Victorian styles never reached such lofty heights but few of the preposterous chignons and braids seen in antique photographs were the wearer's own hair. The fraud reveals itself through poorly matched colors, differences in texture, and excessive quantity.

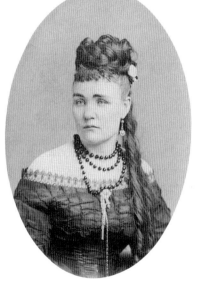

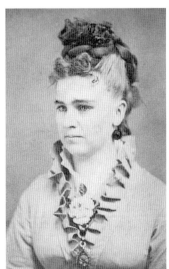

Above and right:
Poorly matched colors and textures are identifiable characteristics of false hair.

Dead women's hair some called it, though in 1867 *Godey's Lady's Book* was pleased to announce that very little of the hair sold in ever increasing quantities was now taken from the deceased. The largest market at the time was Marseilles, which purchased 40,000 pounds of hair yearly in order to produce over 55,000 chignons. Those who couldn't afford costly human hairpieces turned to other materials. Flax, wool, horsehair, and frayed lengths of manila were intermingled with natural hair on American heads at a cost of $2,000,000 per year. Critics were of the opinion that it had gone too far.

"Well, at this moment three yards of hair are the fashion," *Harper's Bazar* dryly commented, watching women pin on high coronets of braids, long sausage-like curls, and larger chignons than ever. "All the charm of a coiffure is lost as soon as one sees nothing but artificial tresses in those curls and bandeaux," *Peterson's Magazine* warned. And the "woman question," according to *Appleton's Journal*, had now become, "Where did you buy your back hair?"

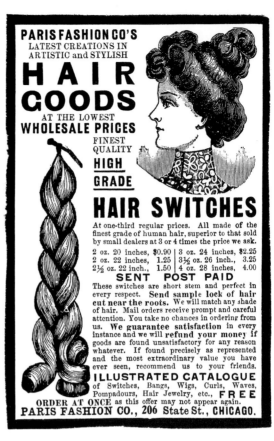

Typical magazine advertisement of the 1890s.

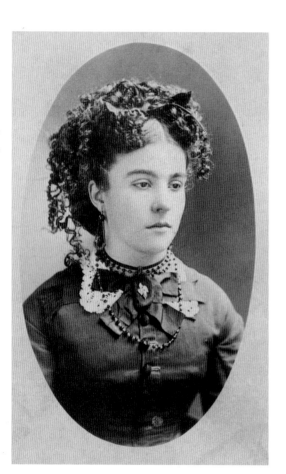

Left and right:
Too much of a good thing could quickly become ludicrous.

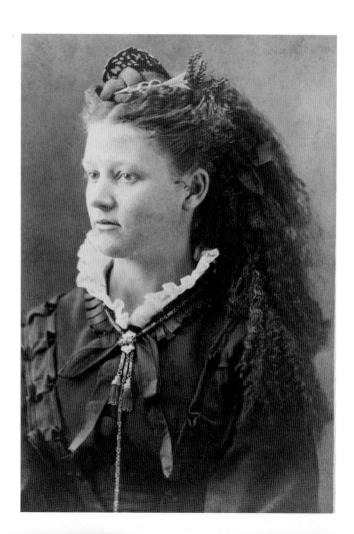

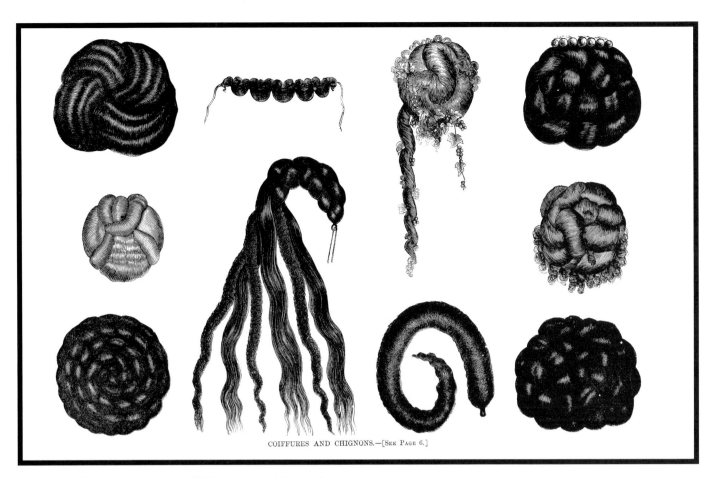

COIFFURES AND CHIGNONS.—[See Page 6.]

Prepared coiffures and chignons for 1867 appearing in Harper's Bazar

"Hair is made to stay in curl by winding it over a hot iron heated by steam. Or by the following method: wet the hair to be curled, wrap it smoothly around a cylindrical stick or tube of proper size, tie it in place, then put it in water and boil it two or three hours; remove it from the boiler, wrap it carefully in a newspaper, and bake in a moderate oven for an hour. Thus treated, it will stay in curl permanently." —*The Dining Room Magazine*, 1877

Keeping one's hairpiece in curl may have been a solvable problem, but a thickly braided plait or switch could hold the equivalent of a full head of hair and weigh a pound, making it difficult to keep in place. Hairpins were vital, as were combs and elastic bands. Even so, chignons tended to slip at inopportune moments. One magazine warned rescuers to lift drowning maidens by their clothing, since the hair was likely to come off in the hand.

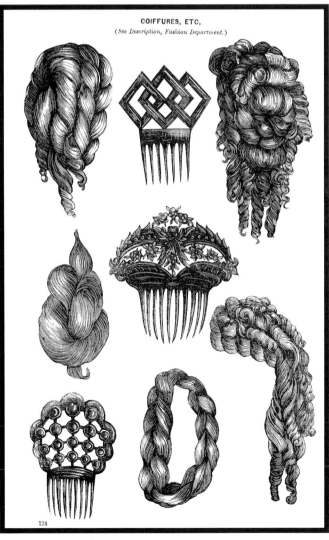

COIFFURES, ETC.
(*See Description, Fashion Department.*)

124

Pre-arranged coiffures and ornamental combs for 1873 as featured in *Godey's Lady's Book*.

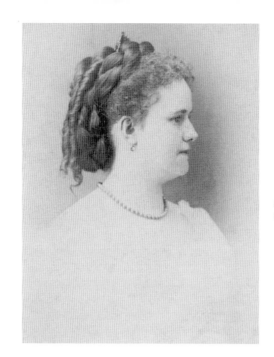

An actual hairstyle with similar additions.

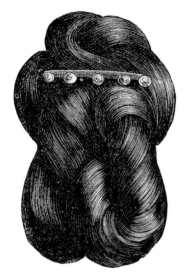

Fig. 4.—CHIGNON.
[See Fig. 5.]

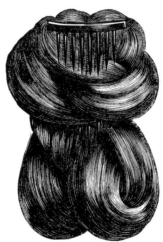

Fig. 5.—CHIGNON.
[See Fig. 4.]

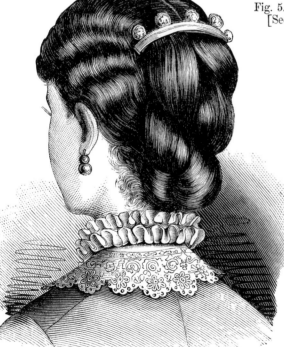

Fig. 4.—COIFFURE.

Fig. 6.
FINGER PUFF.

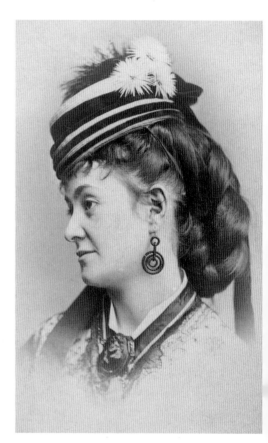

Philadelphia, c.1878-1880
The coiffure such hairpieces could produce.

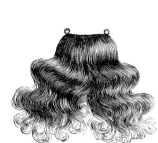

Fig. 1.—Chignon.

Chignons and Frisettes, Figs. 1-6.

The chignon Fig. 1 consists of long and short curls arranged as seen in the illustration, and designed to complete the coiffure when the natural hair is not very plentiful.

Fig. 2 shows frisettes of curled hair arranged on a mull foundation, and fastened under the natural hair above the forehead.

Fig. 3 shows a long waved strand attached to a tortoise-shell pin, and which may be arranged in one or several curls, at pleasure.

For the chignon Figs. 4 and 5 divide the hair, which is fastened to a tortoise-shell comb, into three strands, the outer two of which are twisted and arranged in a falling loop, while the middle strand is looped in a knot as shown by the illustrations. Pin the knot above the two loops, carry the remainder of the strand to the right (see Fig. 5), then underneath the chignon to the outside, and fasten the ends in the knot. A comb with balls of filigree silver is fastened into the chignon.

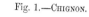

Fig. 2.—Frisette.

A display of available hairpieces from an 1880 *Harper's Bazar*.

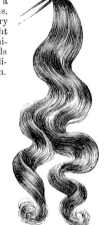

Fig. 3.—Waved Hair.

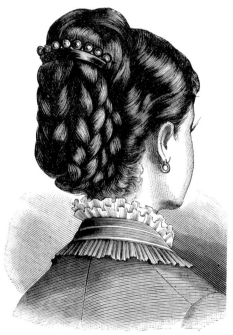

Fig. 6 shows a finger puff attached to a tortoise-shell hair-pin. A number of these finger puffs are fastened under the front or back hair to complete the coiffure.

Fig. 3.—Coiffure.

To achieve the appearance of a full head of hair without so much discomfort, an 1869 *Peterson's Magazine* recommended that a large braid be plaited into many smaller sections, dropped into a pot of boiling water for three to four hours, then baked in an oven. When unbraided it became a permanent full crimp weighing only about three ounces that could be securely wound into a fashionable chignon.

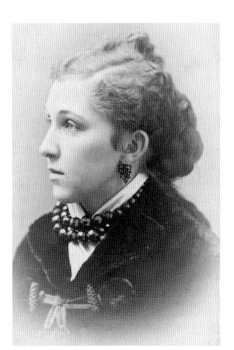

A false chignon that slipped after a day of strolling the grounds of the Centennial Exhibition.

Styles became less complex as the nineteenth century progressed, but the demand for false hair remained high. *Peterson's* reported that ladies who frequented the popular watering places in 1889 appeared at various times of the day with different colors of wigs. To look its best, the lush upswept pompadour of the 1890s called for more hair than the average head provided. Even the liberated flapper of the next century was likely to own a few hair pieces to augment the comfortable but unromantic bob that stood as a symbol of modern life. Never, it seemed, was woman satisfied with what nature had supplied, and the history of her hairstyles became inextricably tangled with all manner of small deceptions.

Chapter Two
All the Rage

Women's Hair: Introduction

Women have always known that a hairstyle speaks eloquently of its wearer. Hair was considered so much a part of the soul in the past that snippets of it were treasured throughout lifetimes, and strands were intricately braided and woven into jewelry. "Hair is as lasting as love," *Godey's* said in 1867. The woman of fashion agreed, and strove to make hers memorable enough to create at least a lasting impression.

But not all hairstyles are created equal. Some women possess a talent for arrangement that others do not, along with the financial means to stay perfectly in vogue. It wasn't until the publication of the first domestic lady's journal in the 1830s that the opportunity to stay abreast of the latest trends reached the average American. *Godey's Lady's Book*, followed by *Peterson's Magazine* and a host of other such periodicals showed even the most remote of rural housewives what was all the rage in Europe—and she happily set about copying what she saw with a distinctly American accent.

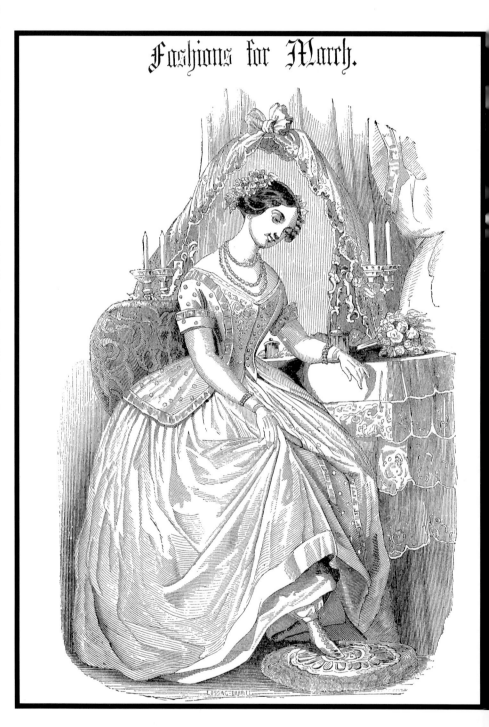

Harper's Monthly, 1852

1830-1860

In 1830 women were wearing their hair *a-la-Giraffe*, lifted high in mast-like bows, fans, rosettes, and other wire mounted shapes made all the more peculiar by additions of false curls, ribbons, plumes, and huge decorative combs. The philosophy of fashion was changing, however, with a sharp turn toward the classical simplicity of ancient Greece. Braids, coils and Grecian knots were adopted, with the front hair parted and arranged in soft curls on the temples. For ornamentation, natural flowers were added, along with pearls, cameos and gold links.

From 1835 to 1840 women turned to their lady's books for descriptions of looped braids, of hair parted in front and turned up behind in bunches of curls, and of ringlets arranged in long clusters at the sides of the head—ringlets to peek tantalizingly out from under the elongated brims of enveloping bonnets. The crown princess Victoria introduced sleek, smooth hair and coronets of braids. Grecian coiffures that were the mode in 1836 were declared out of style in 1838 and revived as the 1840s began. Ornamentation included strings of pearls, bands of jewels, rosettes of gold, lace-trimmed organdy, and flowers.

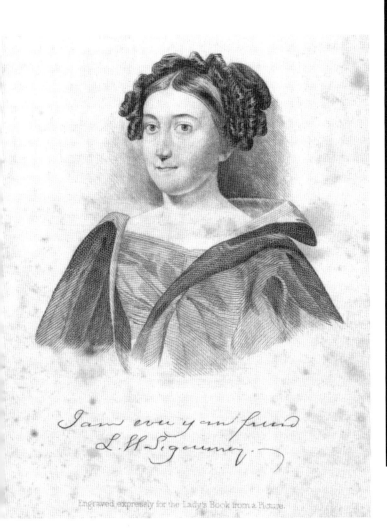

A portrait of New England writer Mrs. Sigourney, done for *The Lady's Book* in 1838.

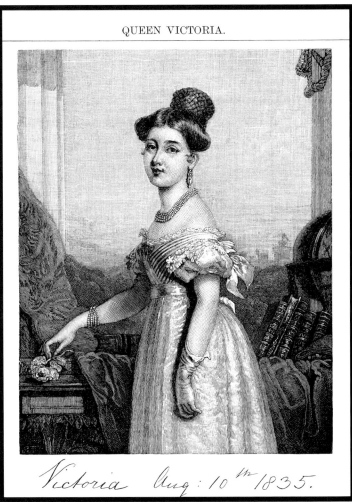

Victoria wore a coronet of braids in 1835, two years before ascending the throne.

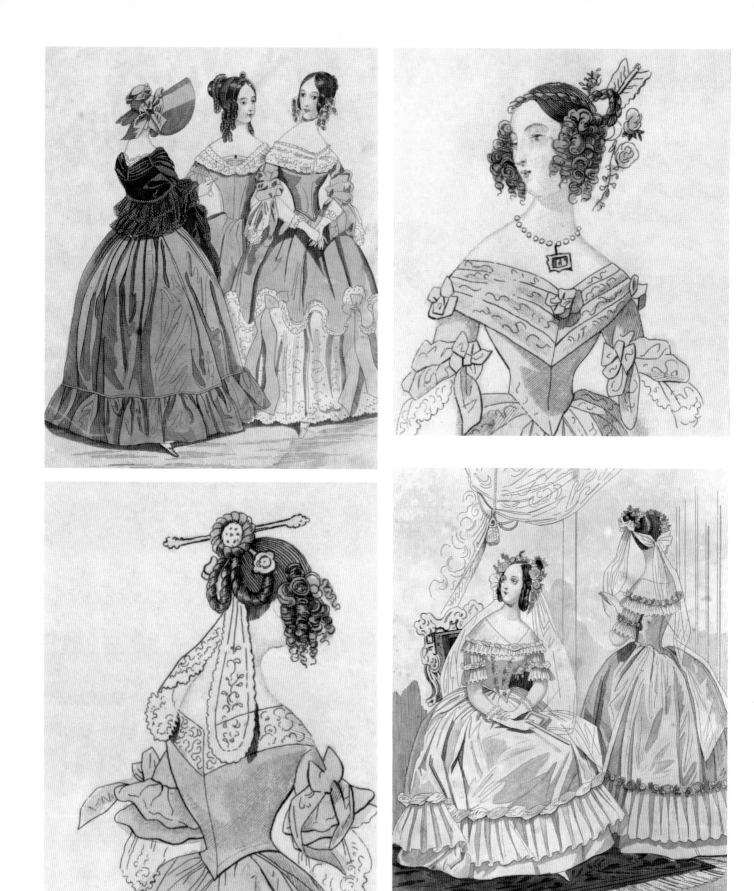

Fashionable styles for 1838 from *The Lady's Book*

The center part was predominant in the 1840s and would remain so with little deviation for over thirty years. Curls continued to be worn but front hair was pulled down in smooth bands covering the ears. Long ringlets gained ever more popularity, while braids broadened into a complexity of multiple flat plaits popularized by young Queen Victoria.

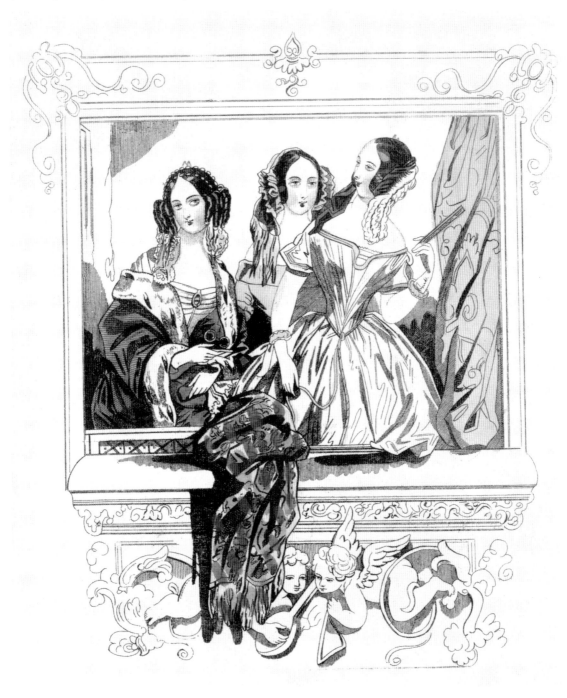

Godey's Lady's Book, 1841
Smooth center-parted front hair and clusters of long ringlets were worn throughout much of the 1840s.

In 1841 celebrity poet Mrs. Norton was seen at a resplendent social affair wearing a diamond chain around a braided bandeaux of glossy black hair. Soon, hair that was growing higher at the back was circled with pearls as well as jewels for evening arrangements. To attain height, back hair was tied off below the crown of the head, combed upward to allow a small cushion to be pinned on underneath, then combed down over and fastened at the nape of the neck. Front hair, by contrast, grew increasingly plain.

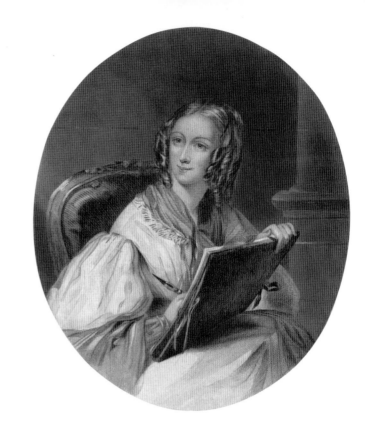

The Ladies' Companion, 1841

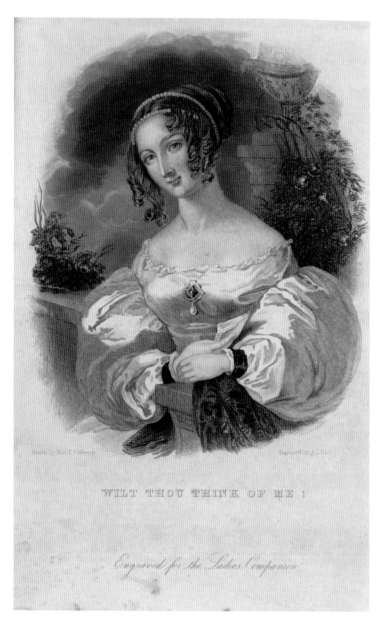

WILT THOU THINK OF ME ?

Engraved for the Ladies Companion

The Ladies' Companion, 1841

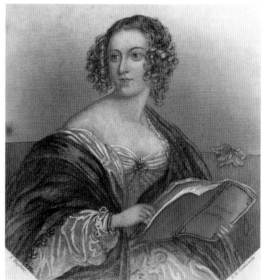

The Parlor Annual, 1847

c.1848-1850
In the second half of the decade hair was center parted and plain, with fullness only at the sides.

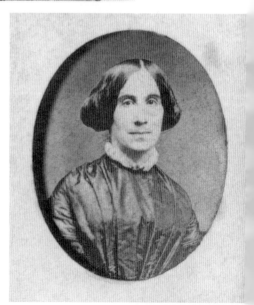

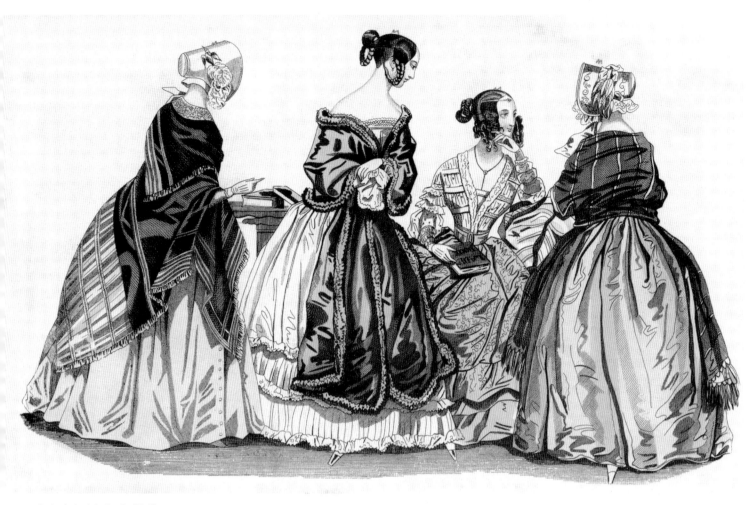

Godey's Lady's Book, 1841

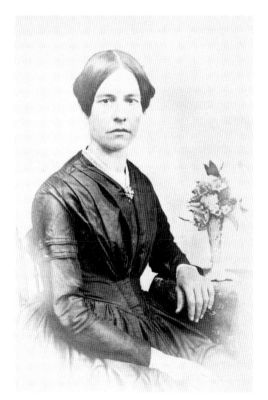

c.1850-1853

FASHIONS FOR MARCH—EVENING COSTUMES.—(*Furnished by* Brodie.)

Harper's Monthly, 1854

15

By the 1850s simplicity had reached the point of severity for daytime while formal occasions called for headdresses of lace, ribbons and flowers to complement the exquisite gowns of the period. Heavy braids were also wound around the head, sometimes topped by a velvet tiara set with pearls, jet or coral. As the decade progressed a surprising new trend was seen, calling for the hair to be brushed smoothly back into a net of silk braid or chenille that later generations would call a snood. *Godey's* provided instructions with or without decorative beads, and hairnets swiftly became an indispensable article of daily wear.

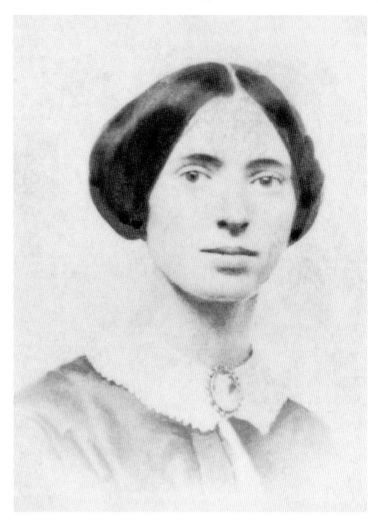

Boston, Mass., c.1857-1860

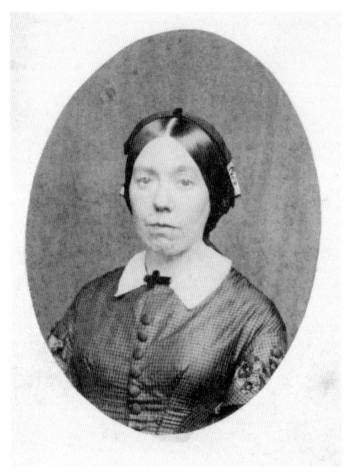

c.1857-1859

Lowell, Mass., c.1857-1859

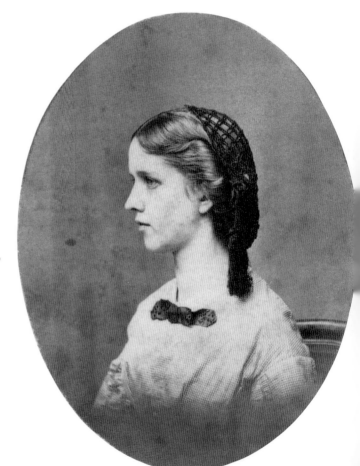

Queen Victoria no longer set the fashion standard as the 1860s approached. She had been supplanted by the empress Eugenie of France, who tied her abundant locks back into cascading curls and elegant chignons for a look that would influence generations to come.

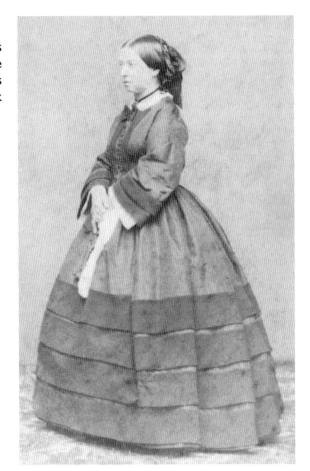

Queen Victoria, c. 1861-1862

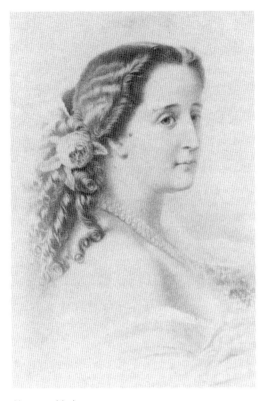

Above and below:
The Empress Eugenie

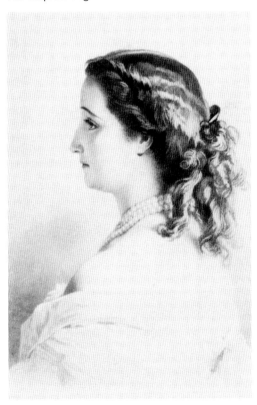

1860-1870

The first half of the 1860s featured hair pulled cleanly back from the face or secured in a net for practical purposes. Braids and coils were added for evening wear with decorative bands of ribbons, flowers, foliage, and the occasional cherry. More and more as the decade progressed, however, the hair itself became the ornament. Imaginative constructions of cascading curls, trailing ringlets, puffs, twists and serpentine coils were built upon and around that marvel of the age—the Parisian chignon.

At its simplest the chignon took the form of the "waterfall." Named for its appearance, this style brought the hair sleekly down over a horsehair frame attached to the back of the head with thin elastic. A net was generally employed to hold the shape. By 1867 the waterfall was under attack for its size and height, yet even more indignation would be reserved for the exaggerated versions of the chignon that came next.

"What a prodigy of ugliness…is the present fashion of dressing the hair!" exclaimed an 1868 critic for *Harper's Monthly*. "It is caprice, not taste, which admires any such perversion of natural proportion as that morbid growth of fashion—the chignon." But admire it women did. And they wore it every way possible from plain to unimaginably fancy, with ribbons and long sausage-like curls hanging down the back.

The front hair was changing as well. "Imagine a row of short frizzed curls over the forehead," *Godey's* suggested in 1867. Women weary of war and the constraints of mourning were ready to imagine anything soft and pretty. When the empress Eugenie was seen wearing light sprays of foliage in her hair...or jewels...or broad braids...stylish Americans eagerly followed her lead.

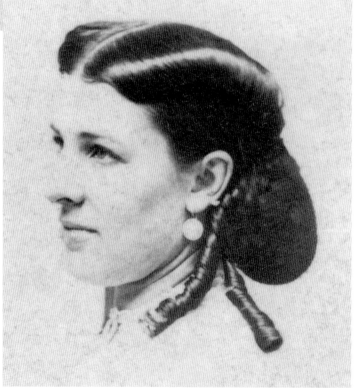

Lyons, N.Y., c.1865

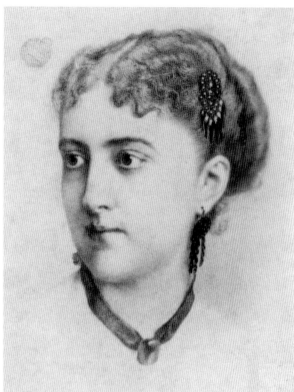

c.1860

Chicago, Ill., c.1860-1863

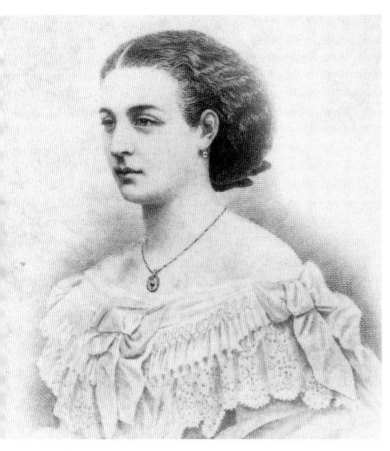

c.1860-1861

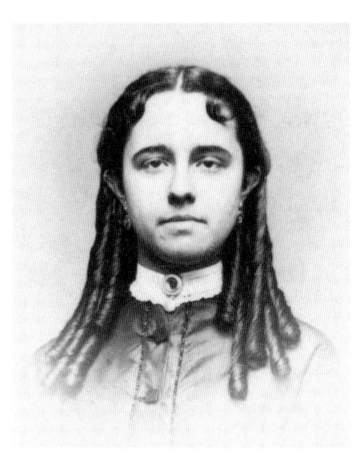

c.1860-1862

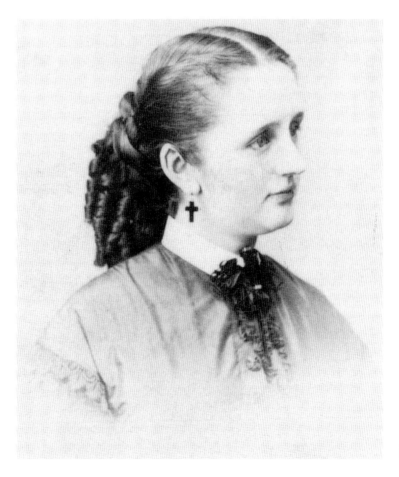

Philadelphia, Pa., c.1862-1864

19

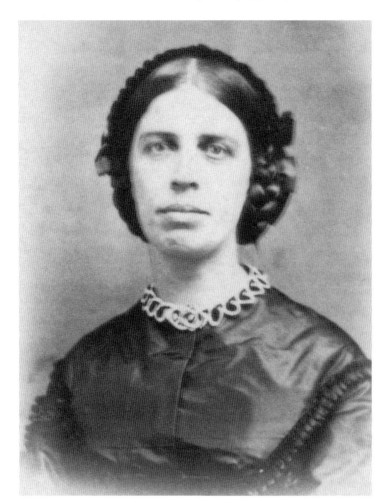

c.1862-1865

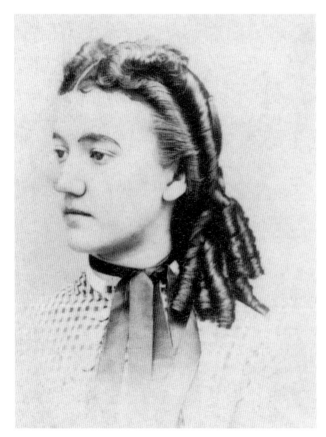

Philadelphia, Pa., c.1862-1864

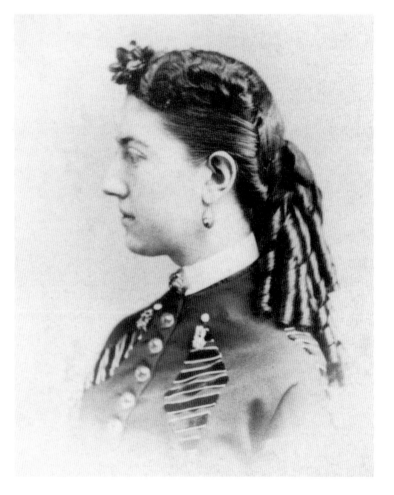

Albany, N.Y., c.1862-1863

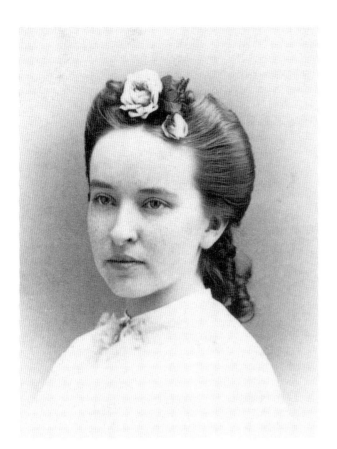

Bristol, Pa., c.1862-1864

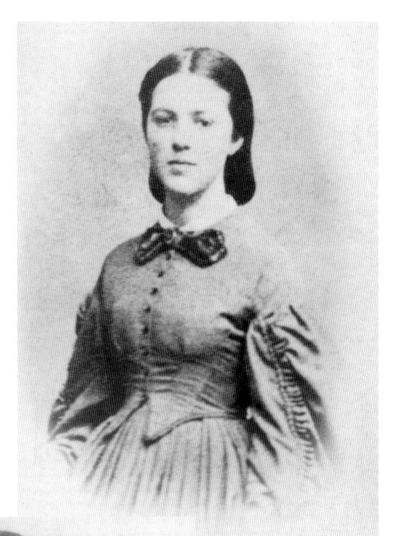

Chicago, Ill., c.1862-1864

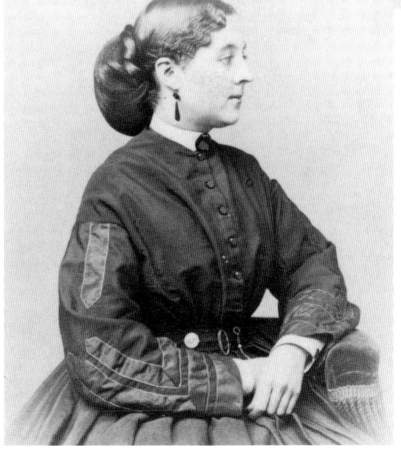

Philadelphia, Pa., c.1863-1864

21

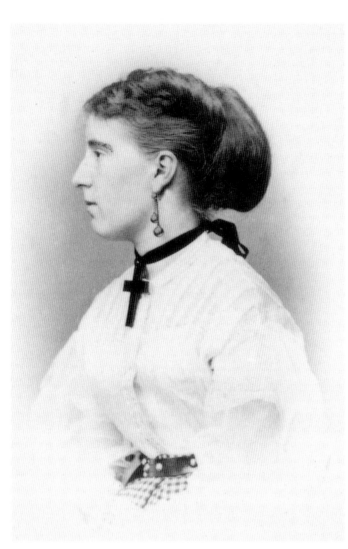

c.1865-1867

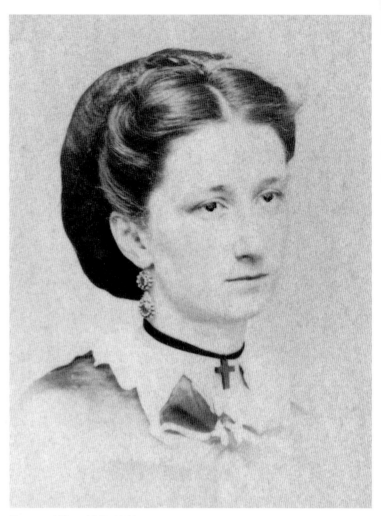

Trenton, N.J., c.1863-1866

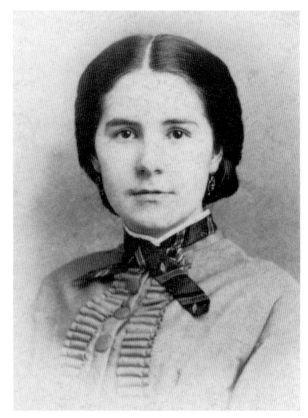

Troy, N.Y., c.1865-1867

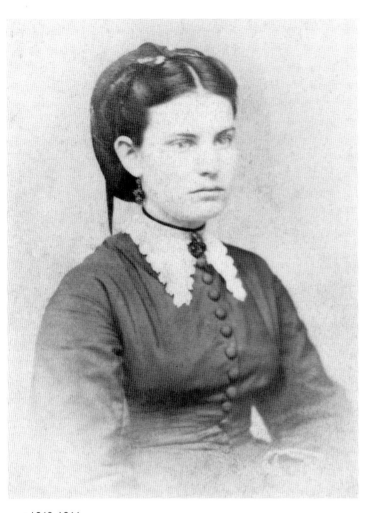

c.1863-1866

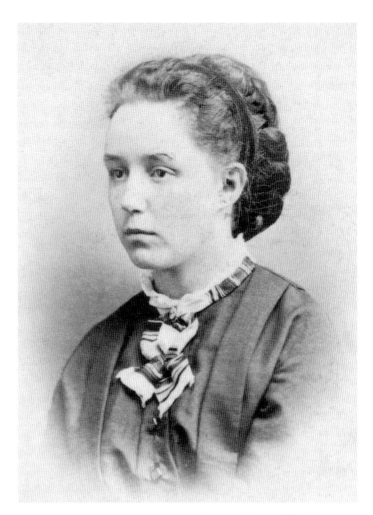

Trenton, N.J., c.1865-1867

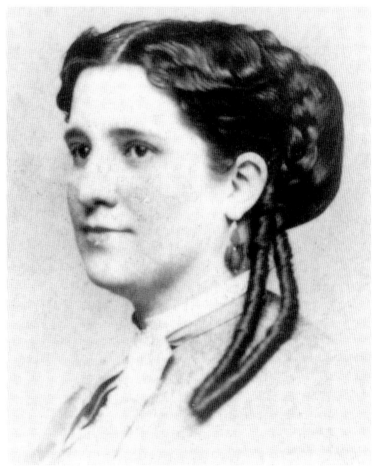

Gainesville, Ky., c.1865-1867

23

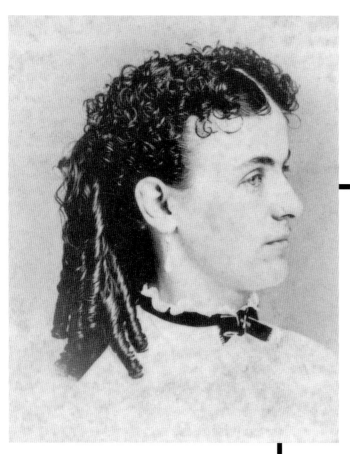

Marion, Ohio, c.1865-1866

DOUBLE CHIGNON

BY EMILY H. MAY.

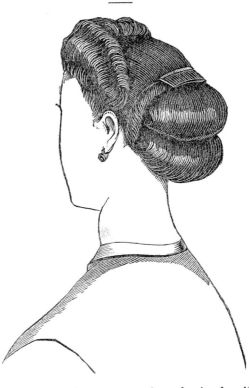

WE give, above, an engraving of a very fashionable Chignon, and below two other en-gravings, showing how it is to be made. Any lady, we think, can make this Chignon.

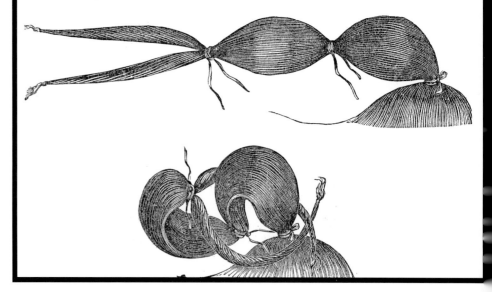

Peterson's Magazine, 1867

24

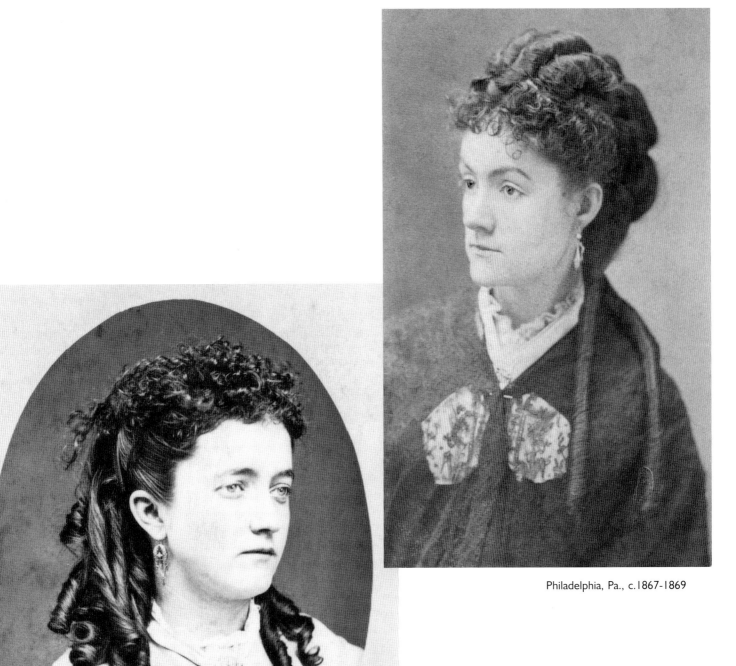

Philadelphia, Pa., c.1867-1869

Jordan, N.Y., c.1868-1870

Hair Dressing.

THESE tasteful and becoming styles of arranging the hair are easily executed. Though they all require a considerable quantity of hair, any natural deficiency may readily be supplied by artistically-made braids, curls, and chignons, which form the most elegant of all head-dresses, and which can be easily made to look precisely like one's own hair.

MARIE ANTOINETTE COIFFURE.—In this, as in all the other styles which we give, a small braid is made of the back hair, which serves to fasten the chignon. Part the hair in a line from ear to ear; tie the back hair low in the neck; brush the front hair upward, and confine it by means of a hoop of shell, jet, or gold; then arrange it in a puff, passing the ends underneath the same. Knot the back hair low in the neck, then carry it loosely upward, and finish with a bow on the crown. Two long curls, falling behind, and short curls in the neck complete the coiffure.

JOSEPHINE COIFFURE. — For this, make of a strand of the back hair a braid on the crown from an inch and a half to two inches long. Then wind the back hair over a crêpé which covers the entire back of the head, in the manner shown in the illustration, taking care to hide the crêpé completely. The

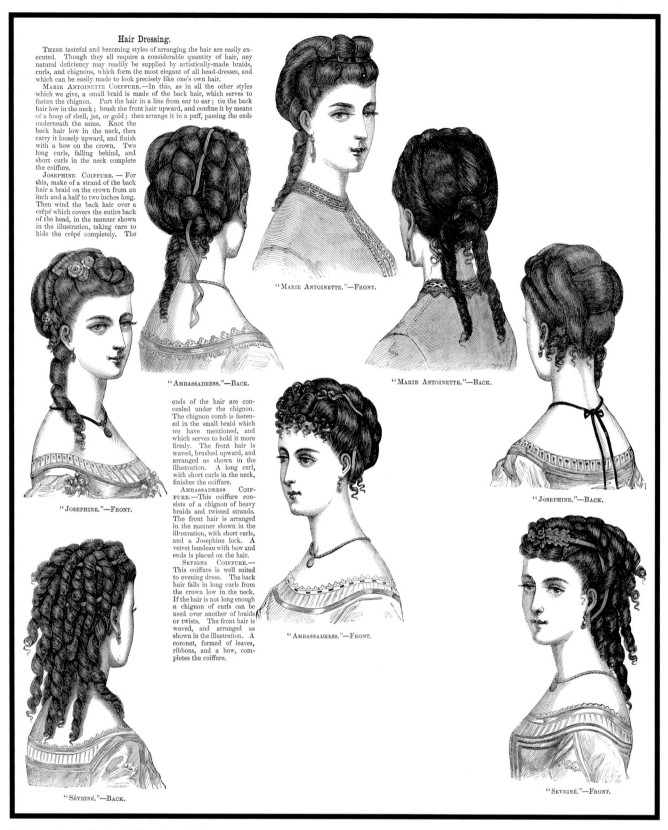

"AMBASSADRESS."—BACK.

"MARIE ANTOINETTE."—FRONT.

"MARIE ANTOINETTE."—BACK.

"JOSEPHINE."—FRONT.

"JOSEPHINE."—BACK.

ends of the hair are concealed under the chignon. The chignon comb is fastened in the small braid which we have mentioned, and which serves to hold it more firmly. The front hair is waved, brushed upward, and arranged as shown in the illustration. A long curl, with short curls in the neck, finishes the coiffure.

AMBASSADRESS COIFFURE.—This coiffure consists of a chignon of heavy braids and twisted strands. The front hair is arranged in the manner shown in the illustration, with short curls, and a Josephine lock. A velvet bandeau with bow and ends is placed on the hair.

SEVIGNE COIFFURE.— This coiffure is well suited to evening dress. The back hair falls in long curls from the crown low in the neck. If the hair is not long enough a chignon of curls can be used over another of braids or twists. The front hair is waved, and arranged as shown in the illustration. A coronet, formed of leaves, ribbons, and a bow, completes the coiffure.

"AMBASSADRESS."—FRONT.

"SÉVIGNÉ."—BACK.

"SÉVIGNÉ."—FRONT.

The latest hairstyles for 1868 in *Harper's Bazar*.

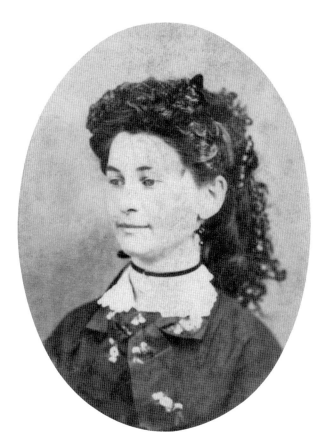

Lewistown, Pa., c.1868-1869

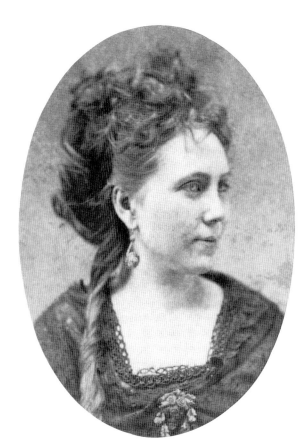

Zanesville, Ohio, c.1869-1870

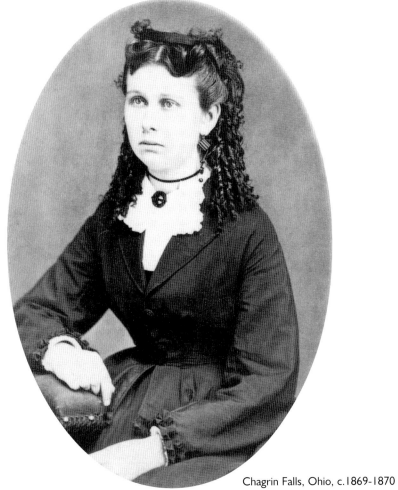

Chagrin Falls, Ohio, c.1869-1870

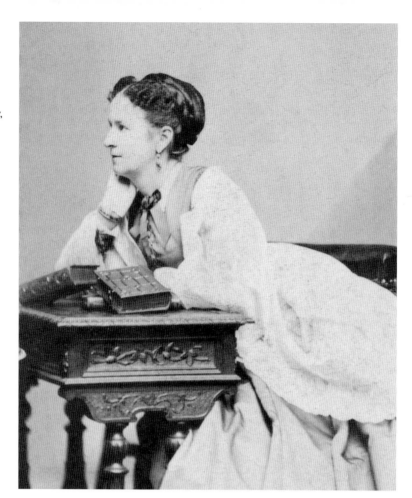

New York City,
c. 1867-1868

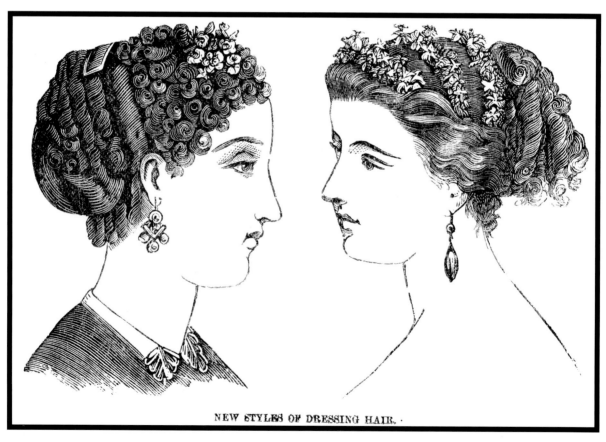

NEW STYLES OF DRESSING HAIR.

Peterson's Magazine, 1867

1870-1880

In 1869 *Peterson's Magazine* had noted the return to favor of the tortoiseshell comb. "The fashionable comb is not only solid, it is very ornamental and very handsome. A very solid comb is, in fact, required to fasten the mass of hair which now forms the chignon." The chignon was not only larger as the new decade began, it was more important to American women than before. Absurdly long sausage curls gave way to looser, more free-flowing tresses. Braids were wound in broad bands around and on top of the head, becoming a distinctive feature of the time. And by the end of the 1870s, the harsh center part dissolved into frizz.

Taken from the name of the French *friseur* who coaxed 18th century heads into frothy confections, frizz referred to thin, short curls that attractively framed the face and added fullness to the style. Long, soft curls were reserved for the back, where *The Dining Room* magazine of 1877 thought they created an aura of elegance falling onto the nape of the neck, and an expression of romantic reverie when they brushed the cheek.

The leading direction in hair fashion was upward, however, and ladies topped their high coiffures with more than just combs. A draping of lace was reminiscent of the exotic Spanish mantillas so admired at the centennial exhibition. Tasteful ornamentation was provided by small jewels, beads, and sometimes a single wide ribbon, while flowers remained as popular as ever—a single blossom tucked into a strategic spot or long sprays of tiny blooms trailing gracefully down over waves and curls.

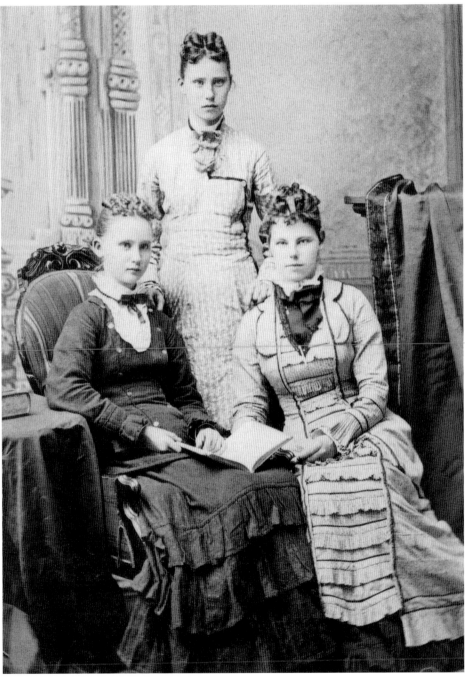

Common styles for the late 1870s.

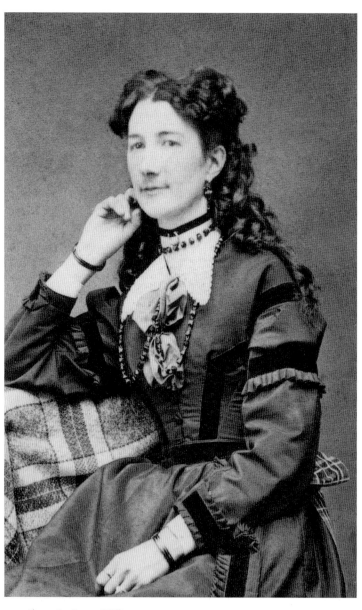

Osceola, Pa., c.1870

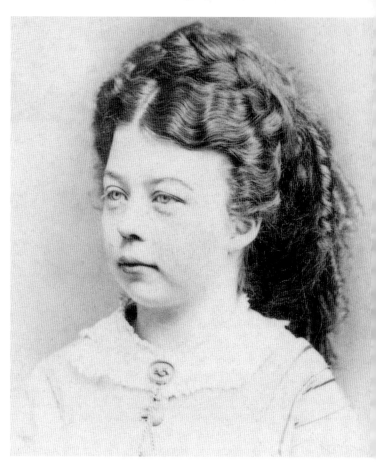

Trenton, N.J., c.1871-1872

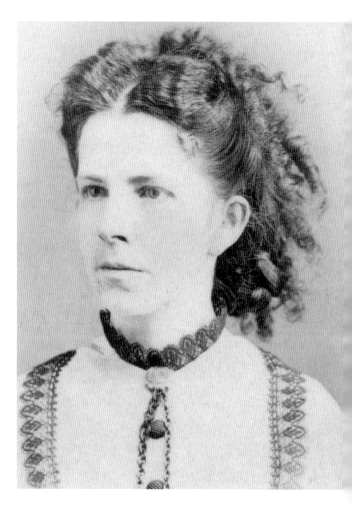

Trenton, N.J., c.1871-1872

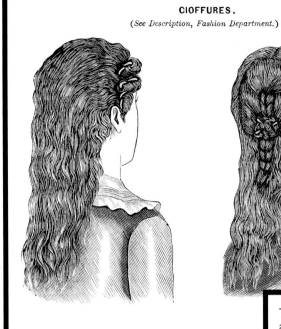

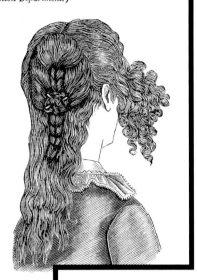

CIOFFURES.
(*See Description, Fashion Department.*)

The latest mode of arranging a fashionable coiffure in 1873 according to *Godey's Lady's Book*.

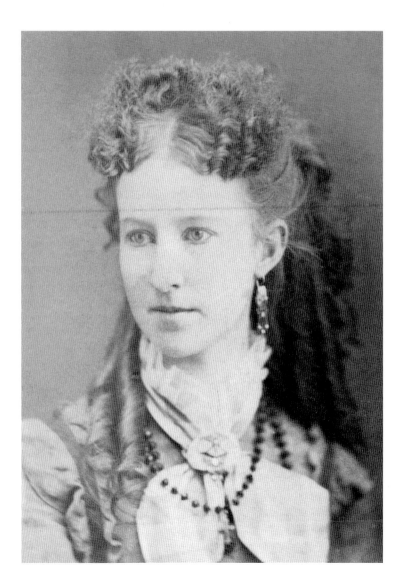

c.1872-1874

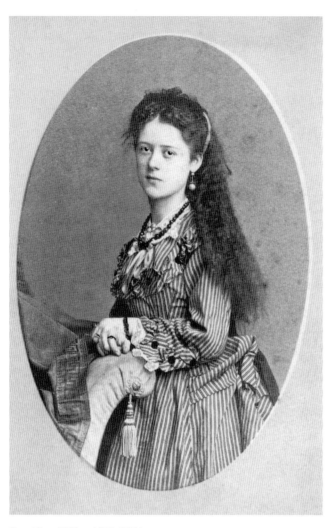

Brooklyn, N.Y., c.1871-1874

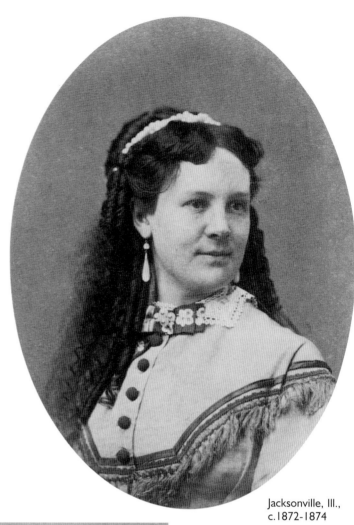

Jacksonville, Ill.,
c.1872-1874

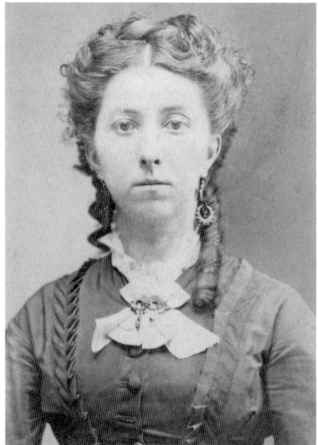

Wooster, Ohio, c.1871-1873

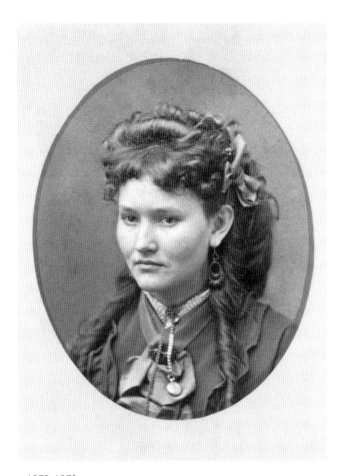

c.1872-1873

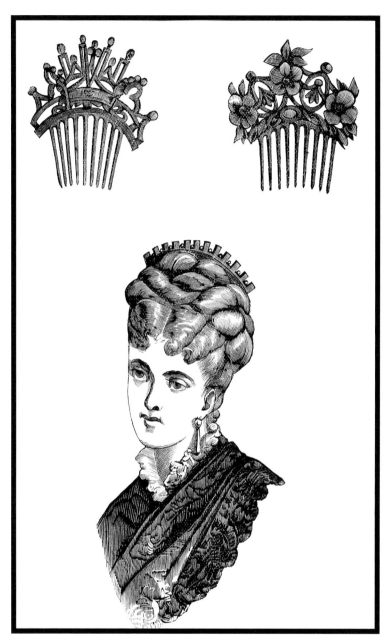

Peterson's Magazine, 1873

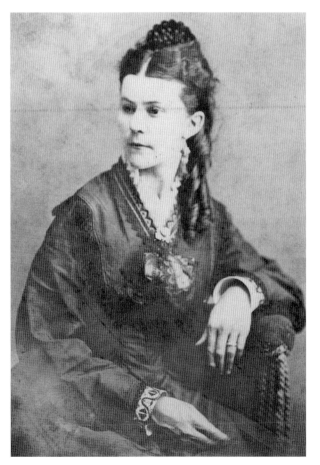

c.1871-1873

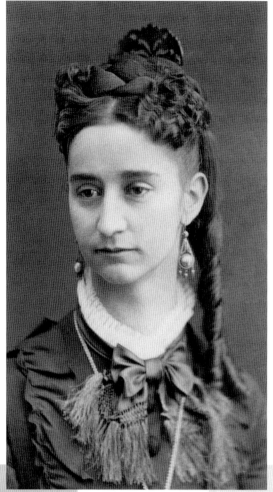

c.1872-1873

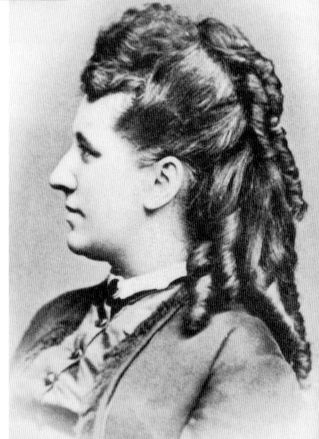

Madison, Wis., c.1873-1874

Boston, Mass., c.1871-1874

34

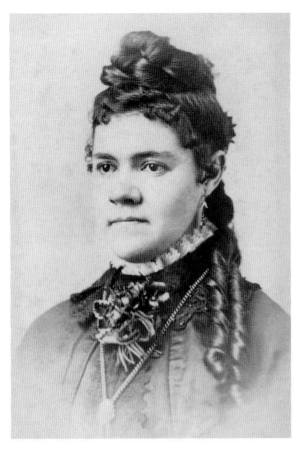

Springfield, Ohio, c.1873-1874

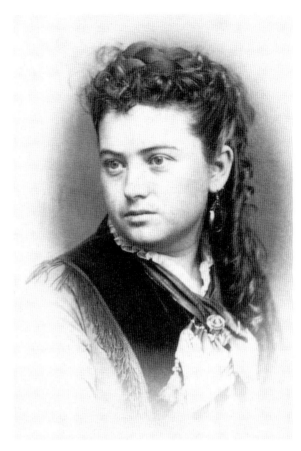

Factory Point, Vt., c.1873-1874

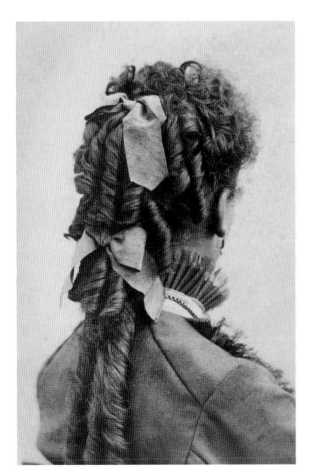

Elgin, Ill., c.1873-1874

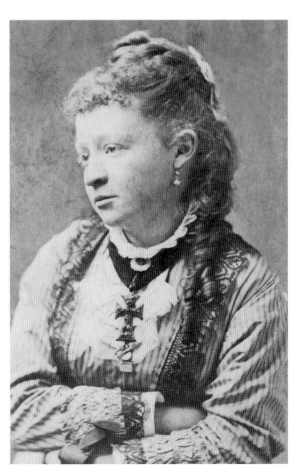

Sinclairville, N.Y., c.1875-1876

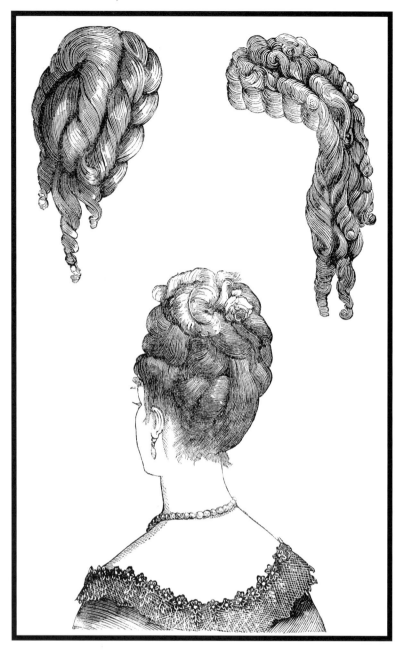

Peterson's Magazine, 1873

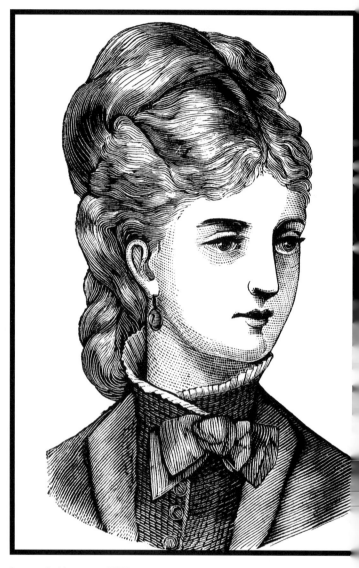

Peterson's Magazine, 1878

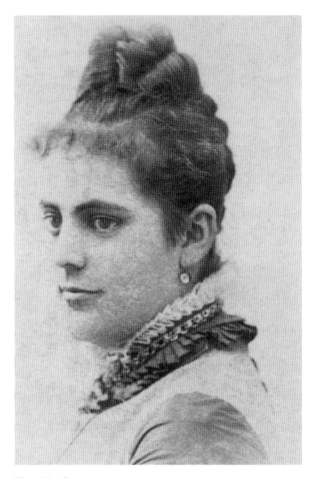

Titusville, Pa.
c.1878

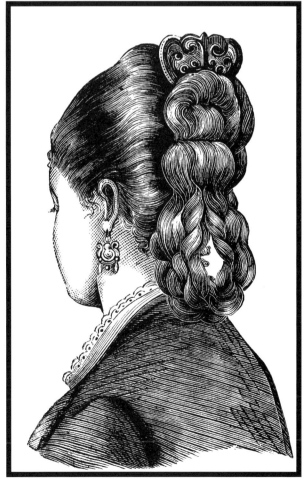

Peterson's Magazine, 1878

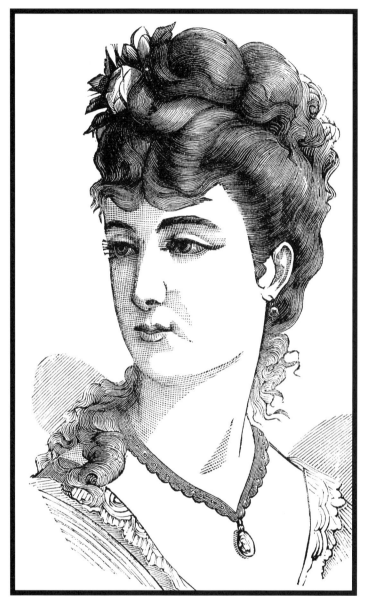

Peterson's Magazine, 1878

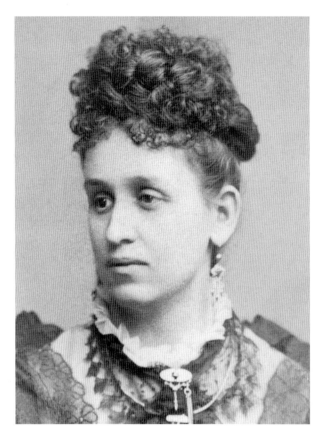

Lynn, Mass., c.1879

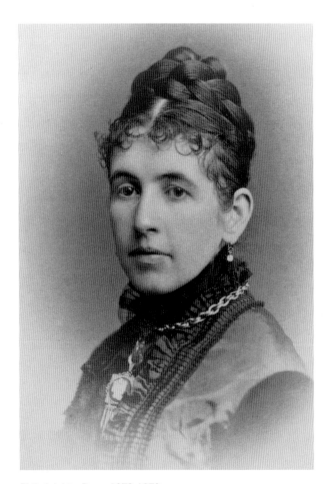

Philadelphia, Pa., c.1878-1879

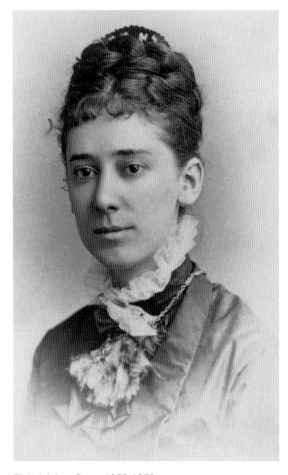

Philadelphia, Pa., c.1878-1879

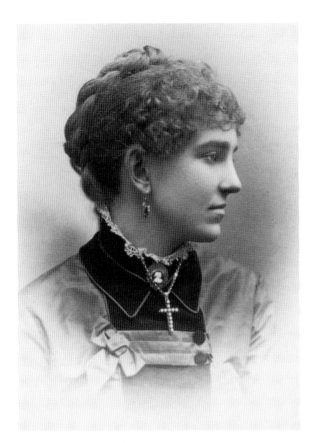

Chicago, Ill., c.1877-1878

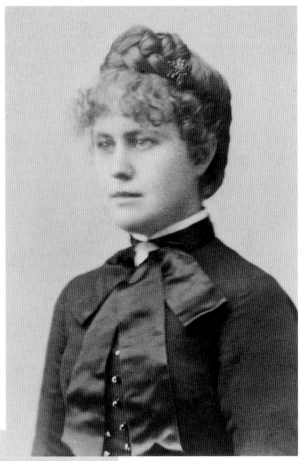

Lowell, Mass., c.1880

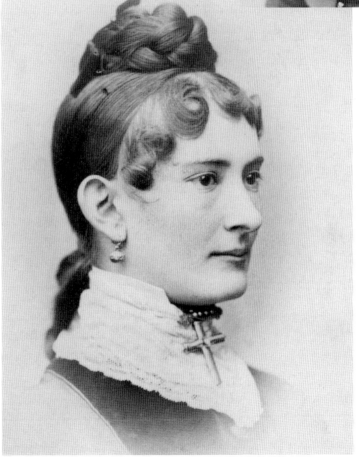

Youngstown, Ohio,
c.1879-1880

39

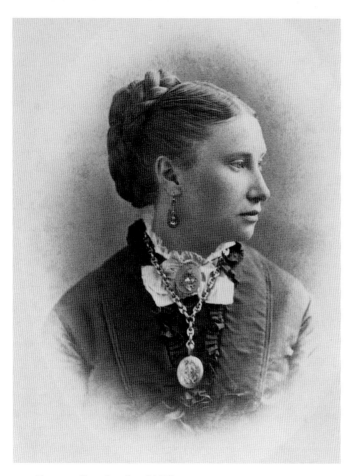

Toronto, Canada, dated 1876

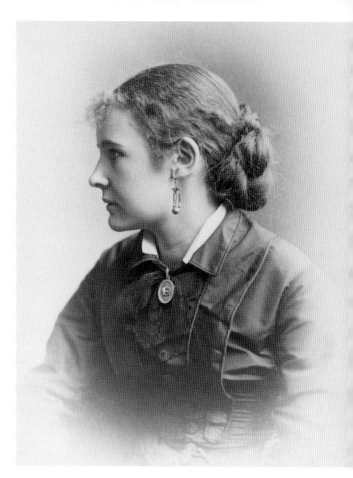

Bangor, Maine, c.1876-1878

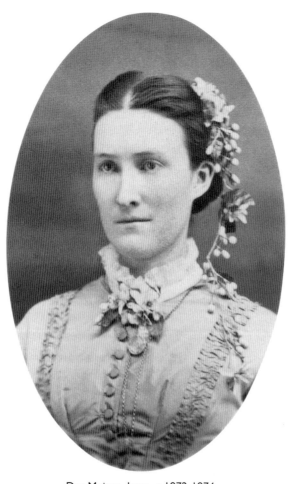

Des Moines, Iowa, c.1872-1874

40

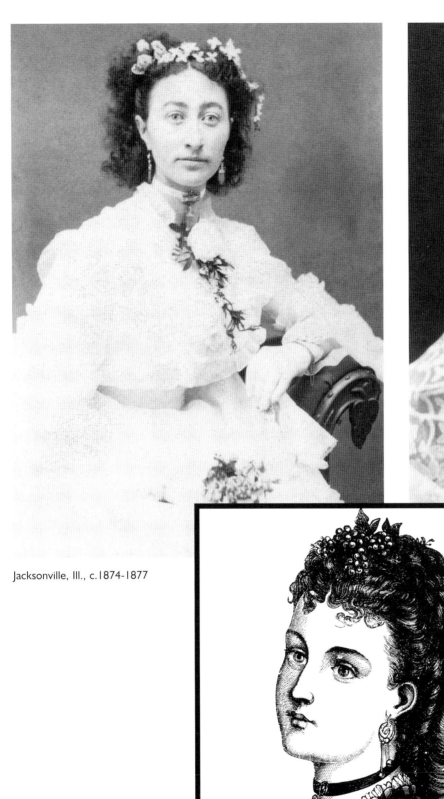

Jacksonville, Ill., c.1874-1877

Champaign, Ill., c. 1877-1878

Harper's Bazar, 1872

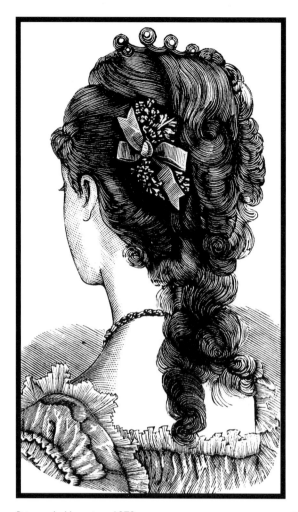

Peterson's Magazine, 1878

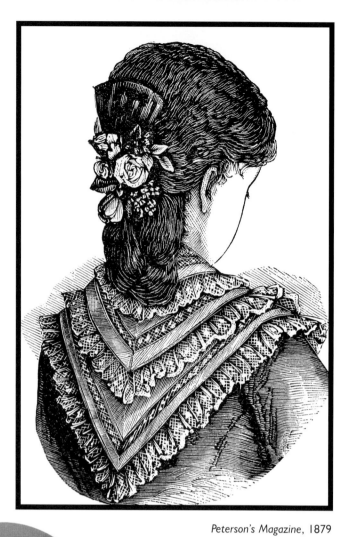

Peterson's Magazine, 1879

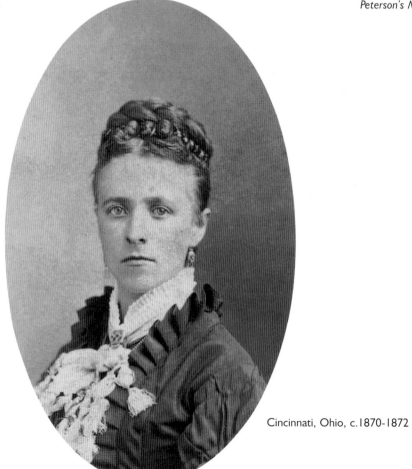

Cincinnati, Ohio, c.1870-1872

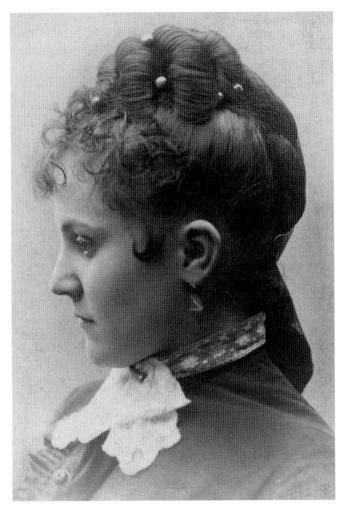

Chicago, Ill., c.1879-1880

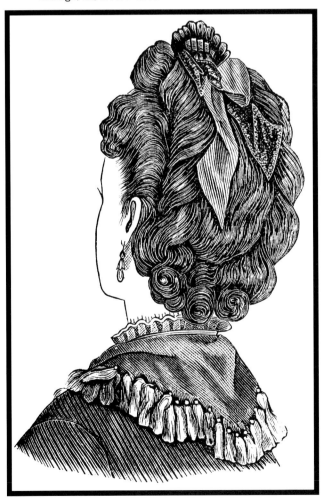

Godey's Lady's Book, 1873.

Union City, Pa., c.1870-1873

43

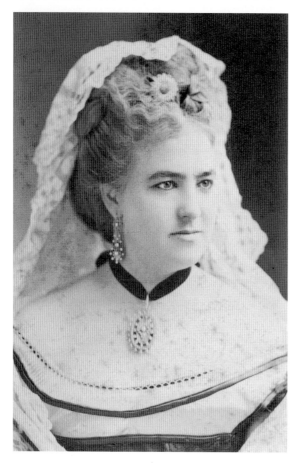

New York City,
c.1877-1878

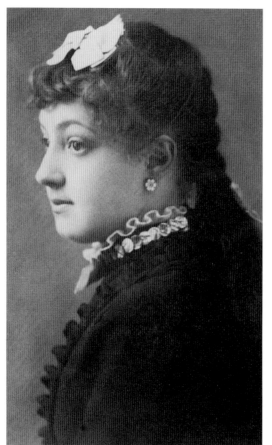

West Meriden,
Conn., c. 1878-1879

Rochester, N.Y., c.1878-1880

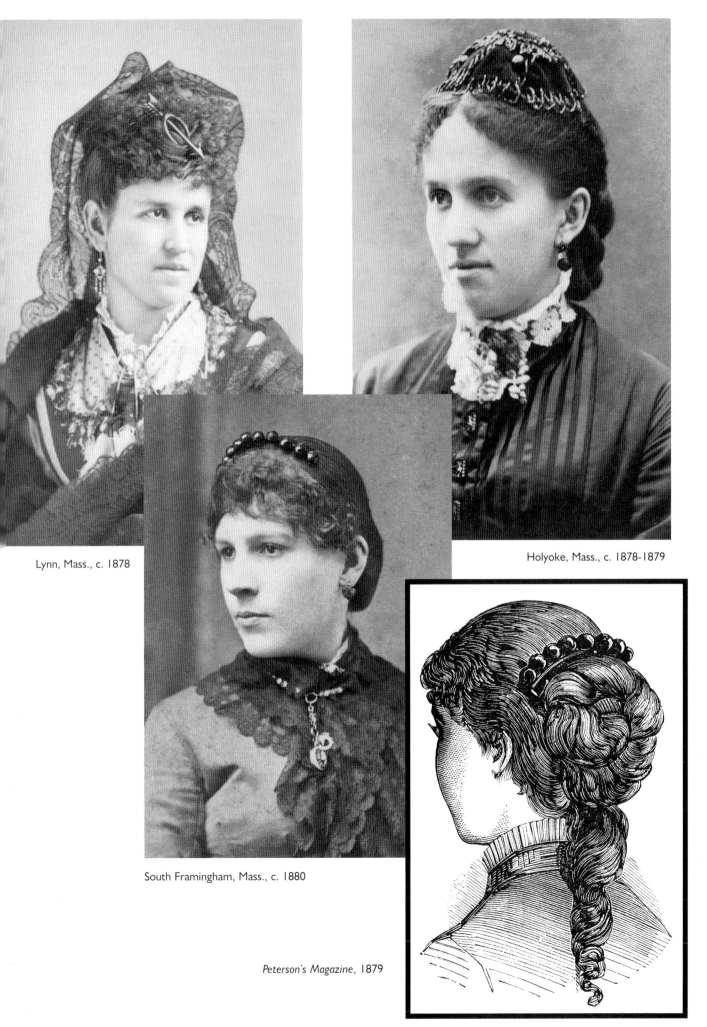

Lynn, Mass., c. 1878

Holyoke, Mass., c. 1878-1879

South Framingham, Mass., c. 1880

Peterson's Magazine, 1879

45

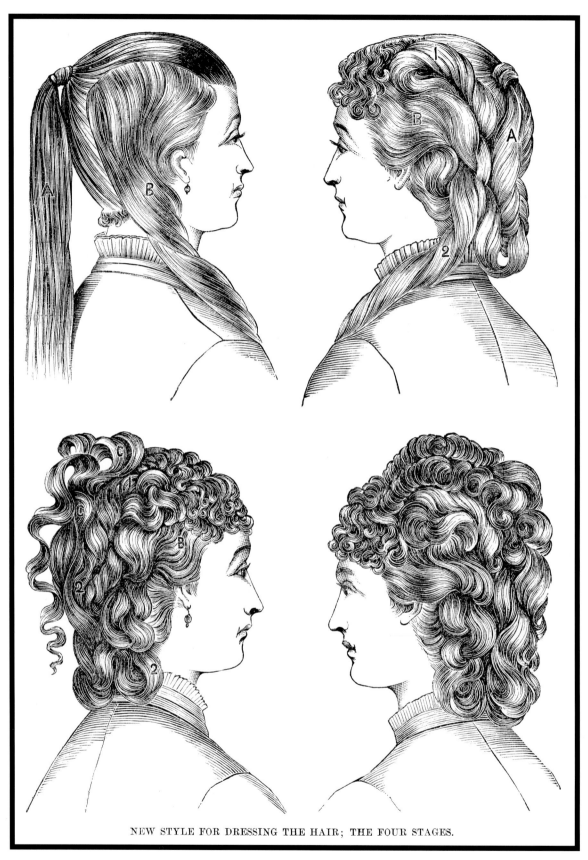

NEW STYLE FOR DRESSING THE HAIR; THE FOUR STAGES.

Peterson's Magazine, 1879
Preparing a hairstyle to take the wearer into the next decade.

1880-1890

"No matter how you dress your hair—pompadour, coiled high on the head or low on the neck, French twist or in puffs…" began an 1883 advertisement for a braided wire foundation roll. It was an effective list of the major styles of the day. The younger woman might allow her hair to fall loose down the back but the mature lady turned, coiled and twisted hers in any number of ways requiring both length and volume.

The newest option was the French twist, fastened in place by a comb, with a blossom or two at the side for evening. Another look growing in popularity called for the hair to be divided in half lengthwise, given a turn, then wound in opposite directions around the head where it could be fastened at the top with an *aigrette*—a small plume of curled ribbons, feathers or jewels. High finger puffs were worn with a side comb or lace butterfly, and the Grecian coil made a graceful return. For less formal occasions hair was often pulled back into low, loose arrangements.

Though the young sometimes retained the straight bangs of girlhood, most women fixed the front in short soft curls the "fluffy English way." With the aid of a crimping iron waves rippled down the front as well, and to correct the wilting effect of dampness, the wise woman carried with her a few ready-to-wear waves or curls on pins. By the end of the decade, the front hair was becoming flatter while the rolls and puffs above grew fuller.

It was Lily Langtry, world famous star of the English stage, who popularized the pompadour, named for the antique lady of towering tastes. Coiled high and forward, the modern version was conservative by comparison to the antique original but far more becoming—and it showed the direction of the future.

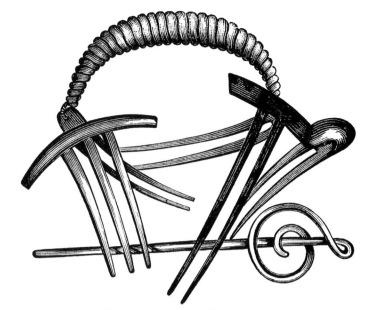

Figs. 1–5.—Tortoise-shell Combs and Hair-Pins.

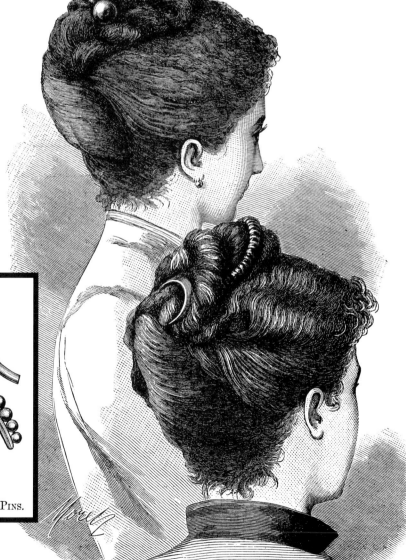

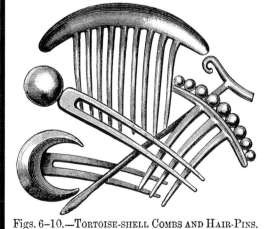

Figs. 6–10.—Tortoise-shell Combs and Hair-Pins.

This whole page:
Harper's Bazar, 1880

47

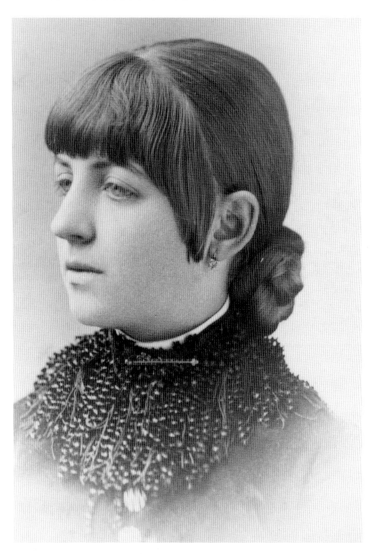

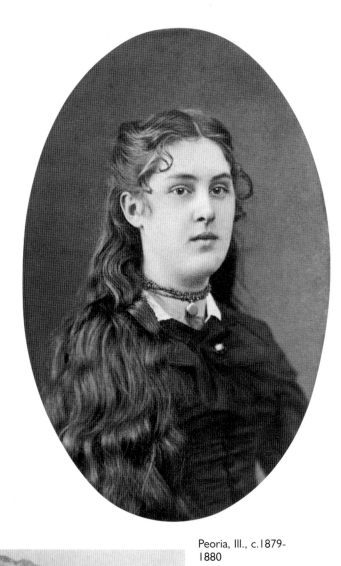

Manchester, N.H., dated 1882

Peoria, Ill., c.1879-1880

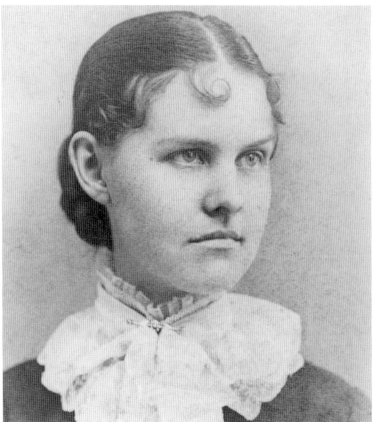

Lawrence, Kans., c. 1882-83

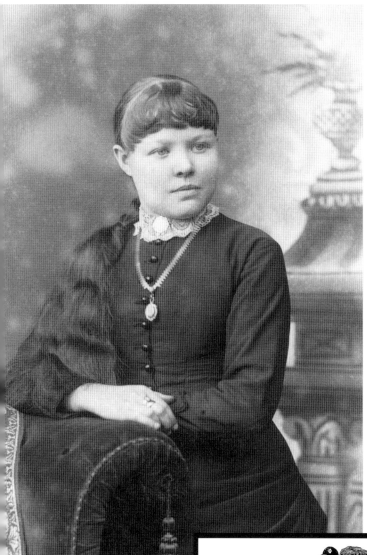

cranton, Pa., c.1882-1884

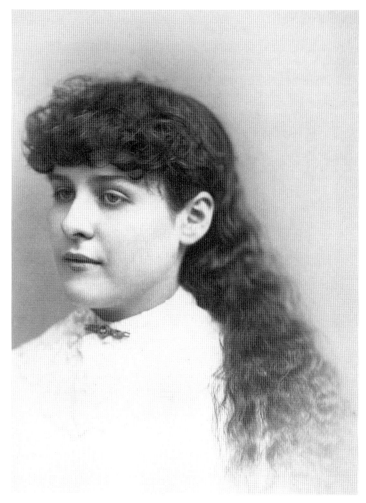

c.1882-1884

Harper's Bazar, 1881
To create this hairstyle the reader was instructed to wave and part the front, then weave the back into a three-strand braid and tie it into a loop. The front hair was "planed" to where the braid was fastened, before arranging it into a puff held with an inserted comb. Loose hair around the forehead and neck was lightly curled with tongs.

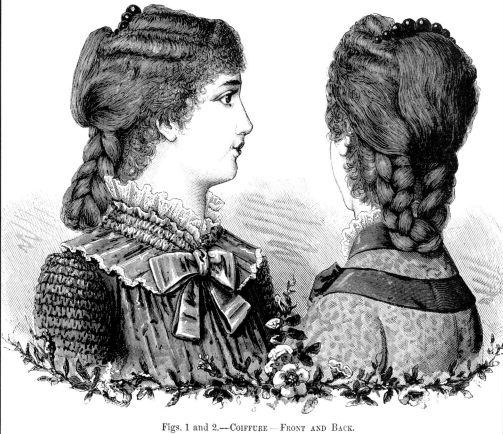

Figs. 1 and 2.—COIFFURE—FRONT AND BACK.

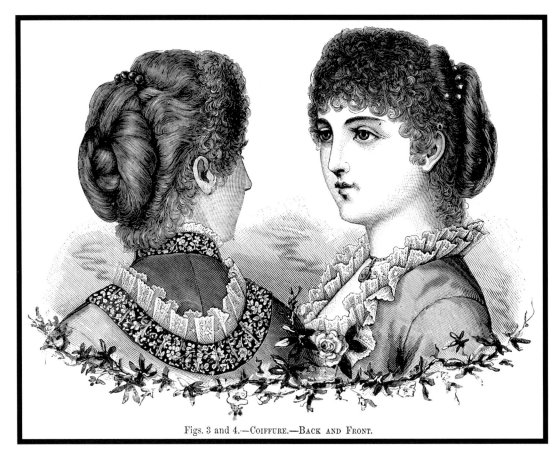

Figs. 3 and 4.—Coiffure.—Back and Front.

Harper's Bazar, 1881
For this coiffure the long back hair was tied off, twisted, and arranged in a knot. Short hairs were curled, then combed out. A ball comb was commonly inserted above the knot.

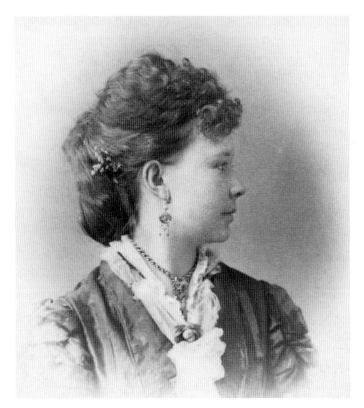

Jacksonville, Ill., c. 1881-1882

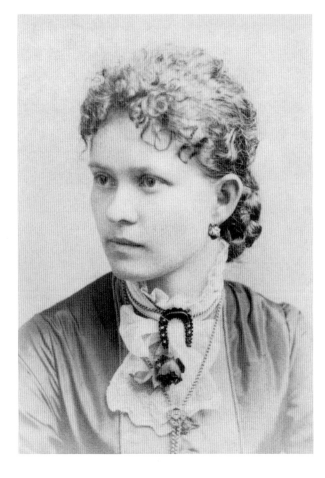

c. 1881-1882

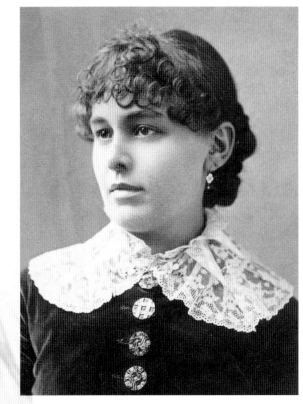

Cincinnati, Ohio, c.1883-1884

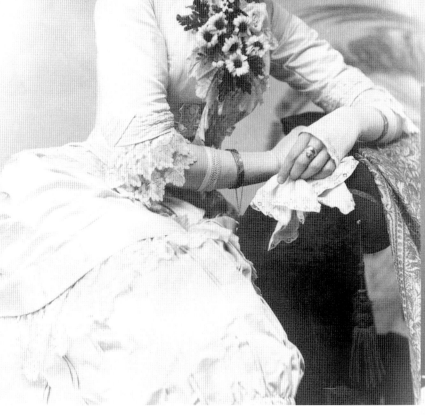

Springfield, Ill., c.1883

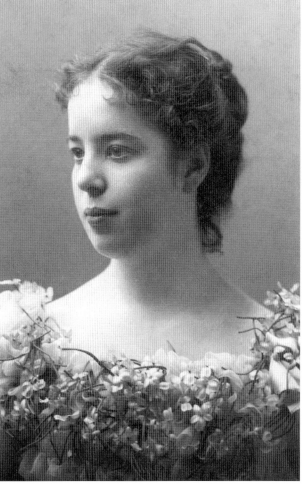

New Orleans, La., c.1882-1883

51

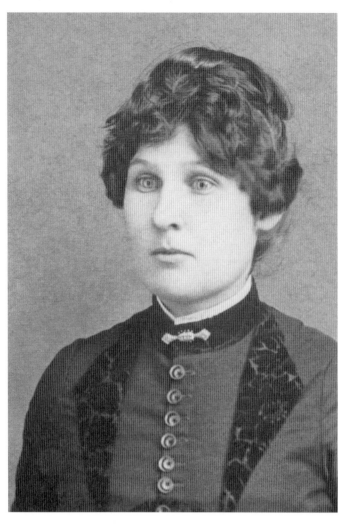

c.1883-1886

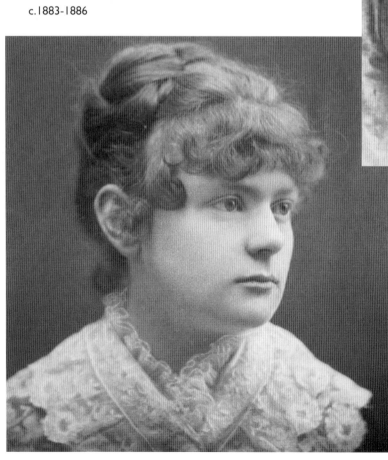

Waterbury, Conn., c.1883-1884

Allentown, Pa., c. 1883-1884

52

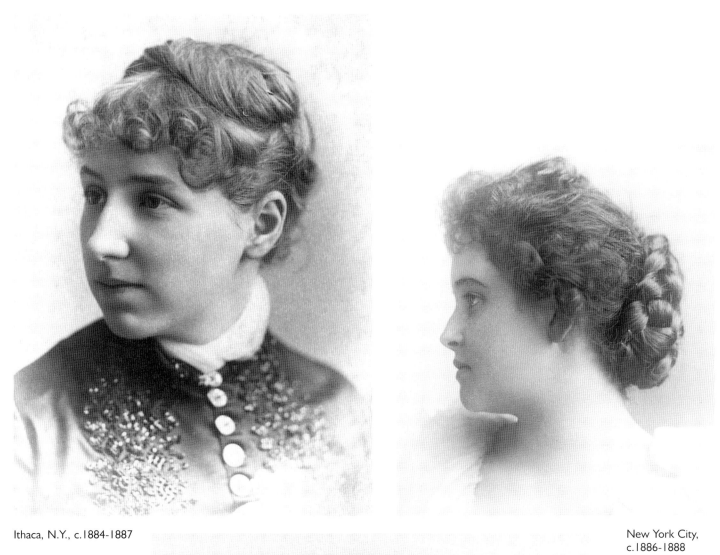

Ithaca, N.Y., c.1884-1887

New York City,
c.1886-1888

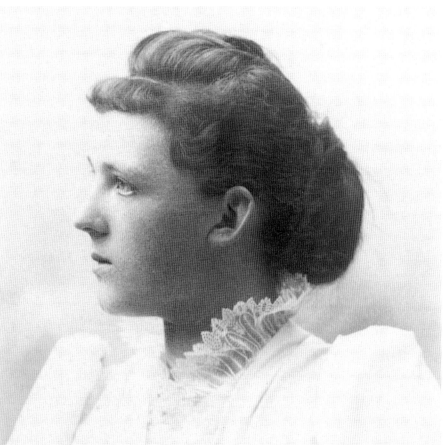

York, Pa., c.1887-1888

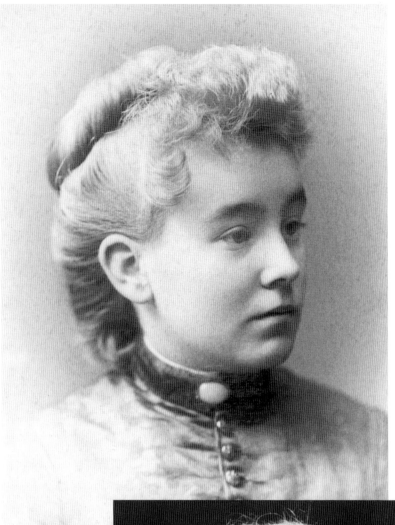

c.1887-1888

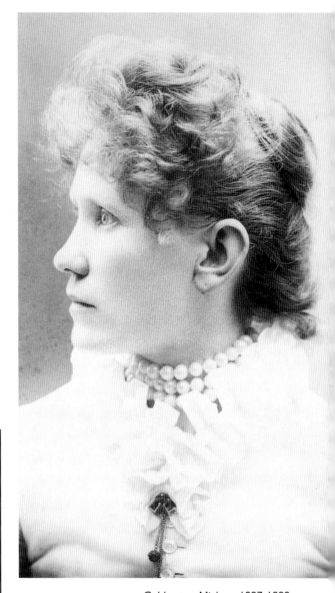

Coldwater, Mich., c.1887-1888

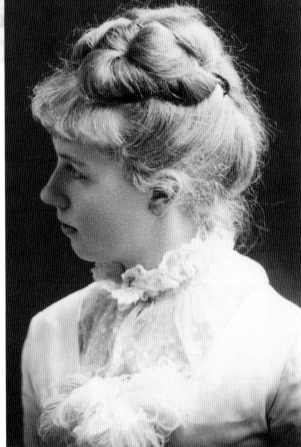

New York City, c.1887-1888

54

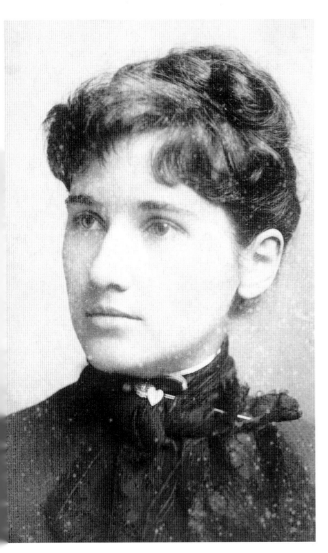

Baltimore, Md., c.1887-1889

1890-1900

"A revolution is at hand as regards hair-dressing," *Harper's Bazar* exclaimed with a burst of prophetic genius in 1891. Even the small details were in flux. "A very decided fancy has arisen for parting the hair," *The Ladies' Home Journal* reported. Parts were being seen on the side and in the center, but not through the bangs. The bangs themselves now hugged the forehead, and the fluffy fronts of the 1880s were considered outmoded in New York by 1895. Fullness moved instead to the crown.

The decade began with twists worn in a variety of ways, from loose and graceful to the tight, constricted form we'd call a bun. At mid-point an elongated version of the knot perched self-consciously on the top of the head, punctuated by the insertion of a pick-like ornamental comb or pin. If the majority of styles tended to look the same, the choice of decoration was nearly unlimited as a passion for hair jewelry swept America.

"It is now scarcely possible to have too many ornaments for the hair," *The Delineator* commented. Carved combs and those set with rhinestones, turquoise, gold, and silver were plentiful, along with high Spanish combs, and hair pins in brilliant diversity. A brief vogue grew for an encircling band set with a small standing egret feather. In notable contrast, a single ribbon was often the ornament of choice for the younger woman.

Compared to the peculiarity of style and decoration that seemed to highlight the decade, the true revolution in hairstyle was comfortable, practical, and deceptively plain. Named for the artist who best portrayed it, the Gibson look was the pompadour reborn with natural, flowing lines that were becoming to anyone, and in step with the needs of the athletic new American woman.

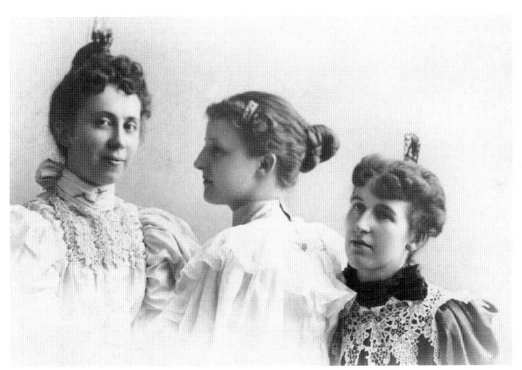

Popular hairstyles of the mid to late 1890s.

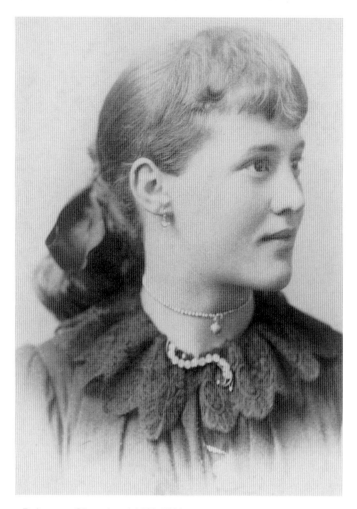

Delaware, Ohio, dated 1890-1891

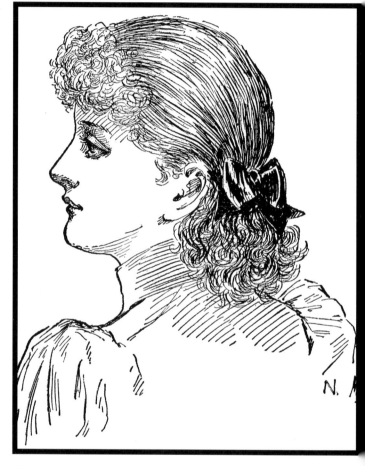

The Ladies' Home Journal, 1891
Sarah Bernhardt popularized this informal style, often worn by schoolgirls and young women. A clasp or ribbon, usually black, drew the back hair together. To avoid a "wooly" appearance to the curls, the hair was dampened with a setting lotion, rolled over a lead pencil, wrapped in curling paper, and pinched with a hot "pressing" iron.

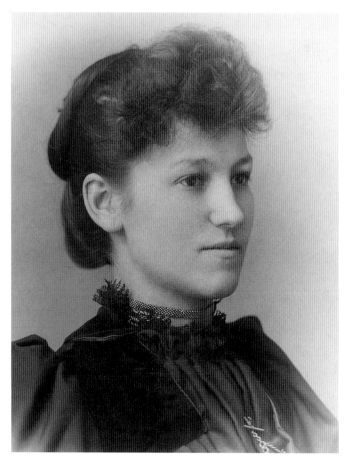

Williamsport, Pa., c. 1892-94

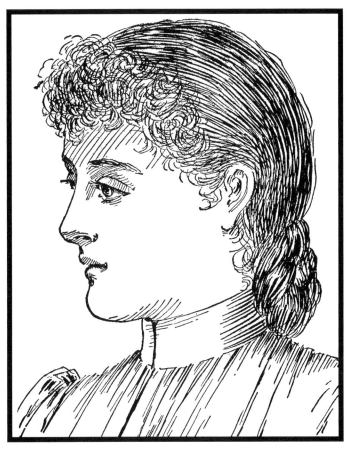

Long hair drawn into a loose knot and fastened low on the neck was described as a look "certain to be approved of" in 1891 by *The Ladies' Home Journal*. A decorative shell pin was sometimes stuck through the knot.

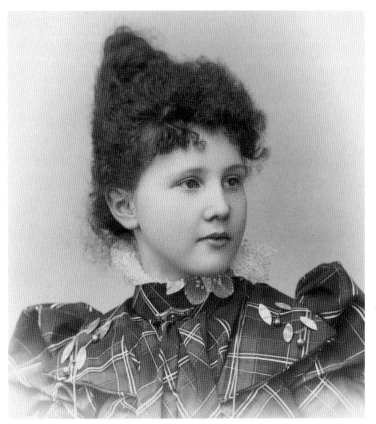

Above and below:
c.1890-1892

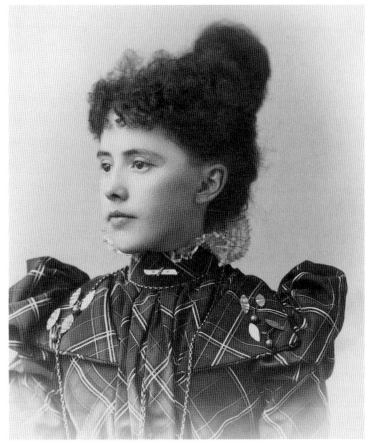

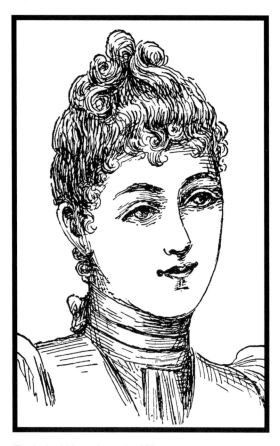

The Ladies' Home Journal, 1892

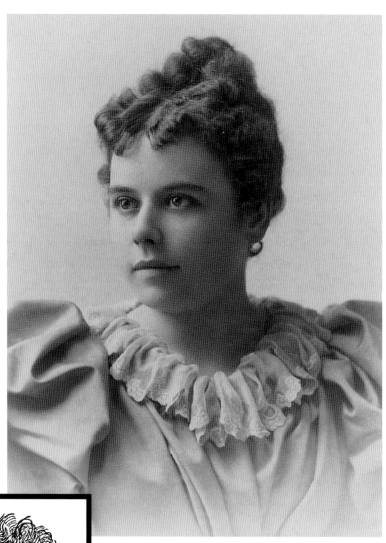

Toronto, Canada, c.1894-1896

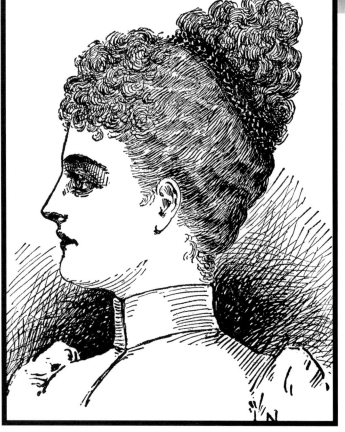

The Ladies' Home Journal, 1892
The return of the Grecian look allowed the woman with abundant hair to build height. She might simply brush the back hair high over the front, or she might build the full Greek extreme. A golden band sometimes circled the arrangement in classical style.

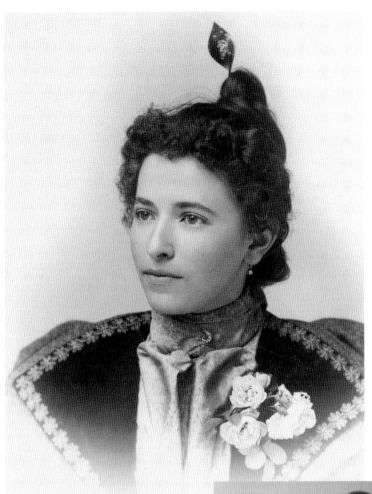

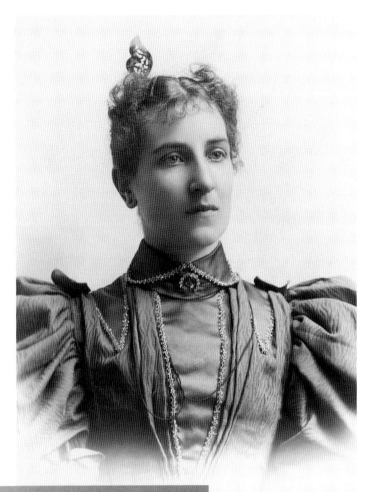

Canonsburg, Pa., c.1895-1898

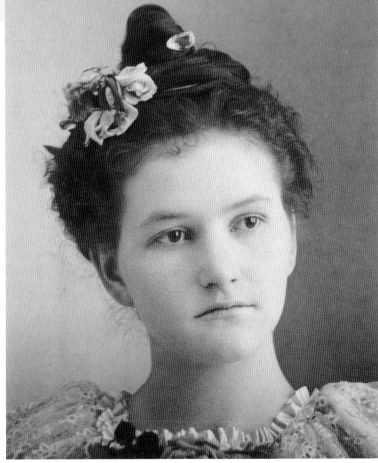

Enid, Okla., c.1895-1898

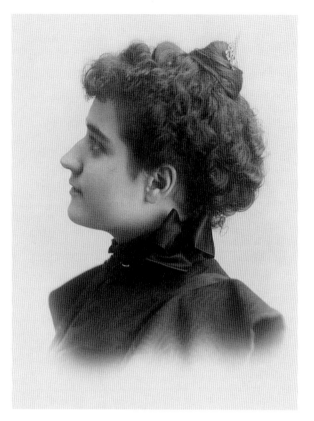

Oskaloosa, Ind., c.1895-1898

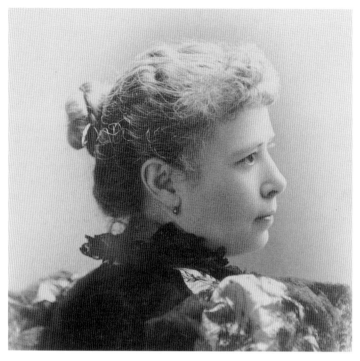

Syracuse, N.Y., c.1895-1897

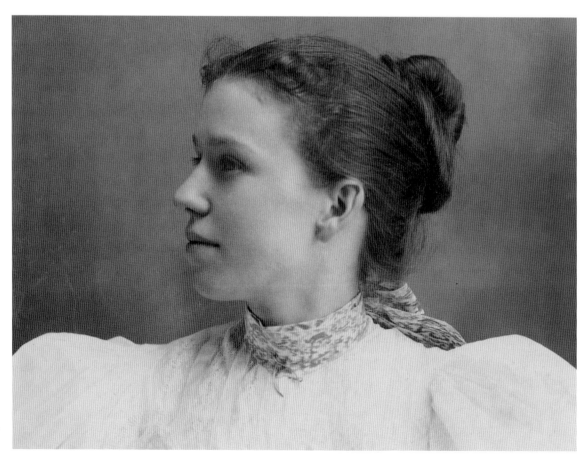

Braddock,
Pa., c.1896-
1898

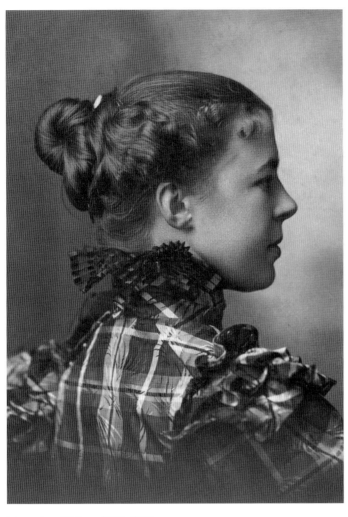

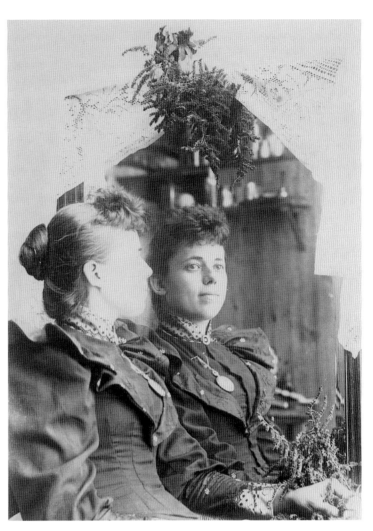

Ishpeming, Mich., c.1896-1898

c.1895-1897

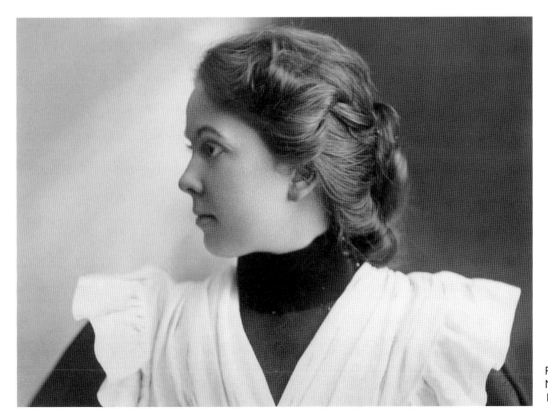

Port Huron,
Mich., c.1896-
1898

61

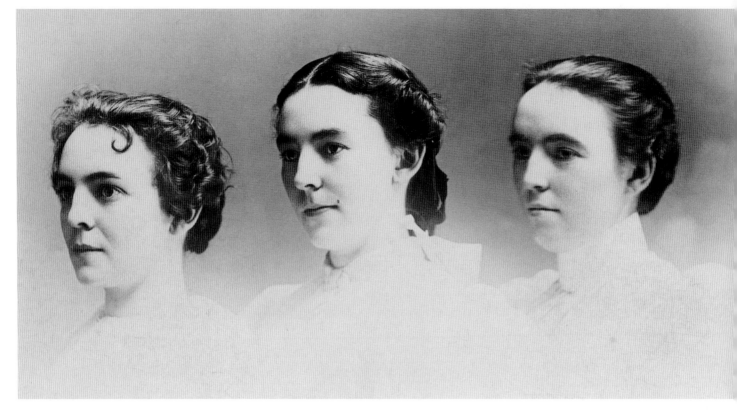

Belvidere, Ill.
Typical daytime styles of the mid to late 1890s.

1900-1910

Charles Dana Gibson created his perfect woman in the image of his wife. He endowed her with beauty, grace, energy, intelligence, and thick, lustrous hair arranged in a distinctive manner that every woman longed to own. The Gibson Girl's hair might be brushed smoothly upward into a coil, or it might rise in a bewitching mass of waves, curls and escaped tendrils, so long as it appeared completely natural, and complimented the face it surrounded.

The phenomena that was the Gibson look did not reign unchallenged, however. Perhaps as a backlash to the rapidly changing modern world there was a brief return to the long, dangling sausage-like curls of the past—one or two draped romantically over the shoulder. A fall of shoulder length hair contained by a large bow produced another romantic look—but only for the youthful.

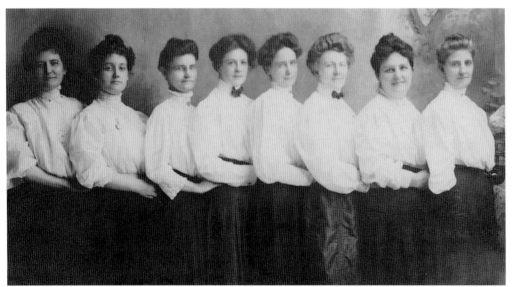

c.1906-1908

At mid-decade the hair began to widen as an accommodation to the enormous hats of the day. Marcel waves circled every stylish head. Parts, which had been missing for some time, returned both at the center and side. Complexity of arrangement also made a return, though by 1910 the younger generation was developing a taste for simplicity.

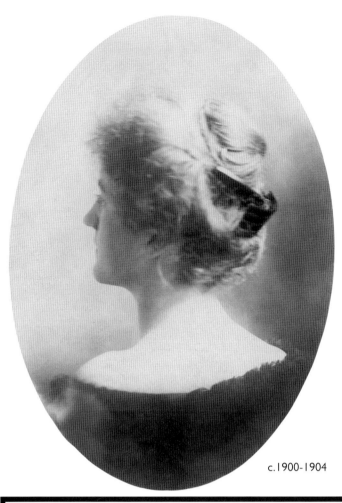

c.1900-1904

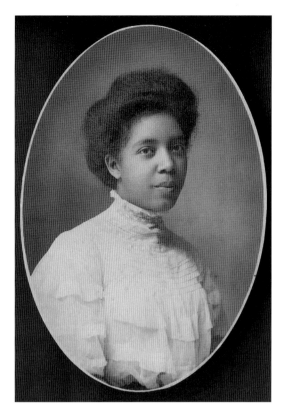

c.1905-1907

Charles Dana Gibson set the standard for the look of the decade.

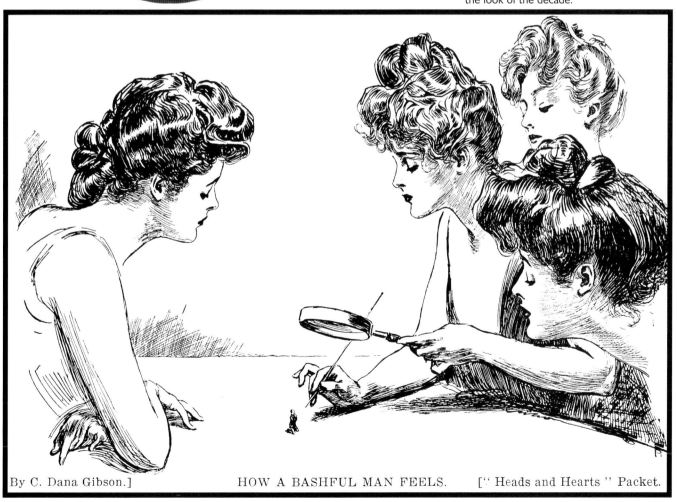

By C. Dana Gibson.]   HOW A BASHFUL MAN FEELS.   [" Heads and Hearts " Packet.

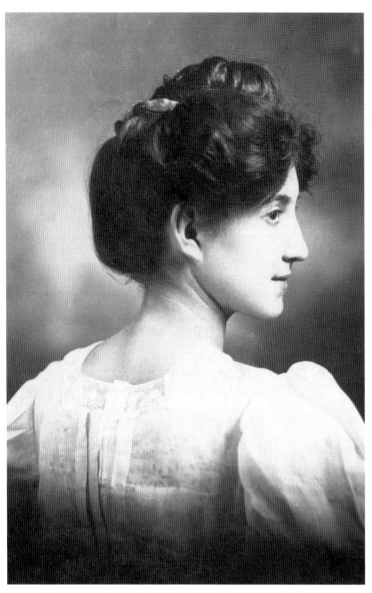

Wichita, Kans., c. 1906-1908

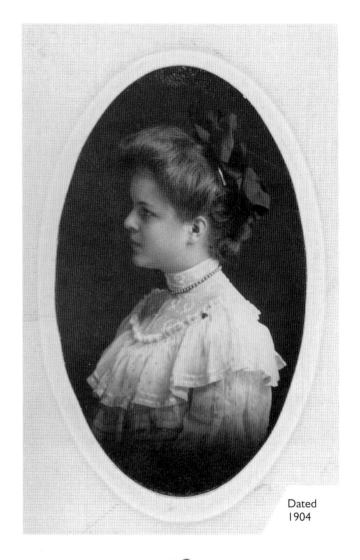

Dated
1904

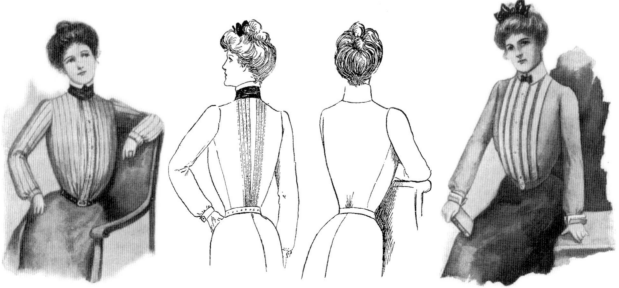

Harper's Bazar, 1901

64

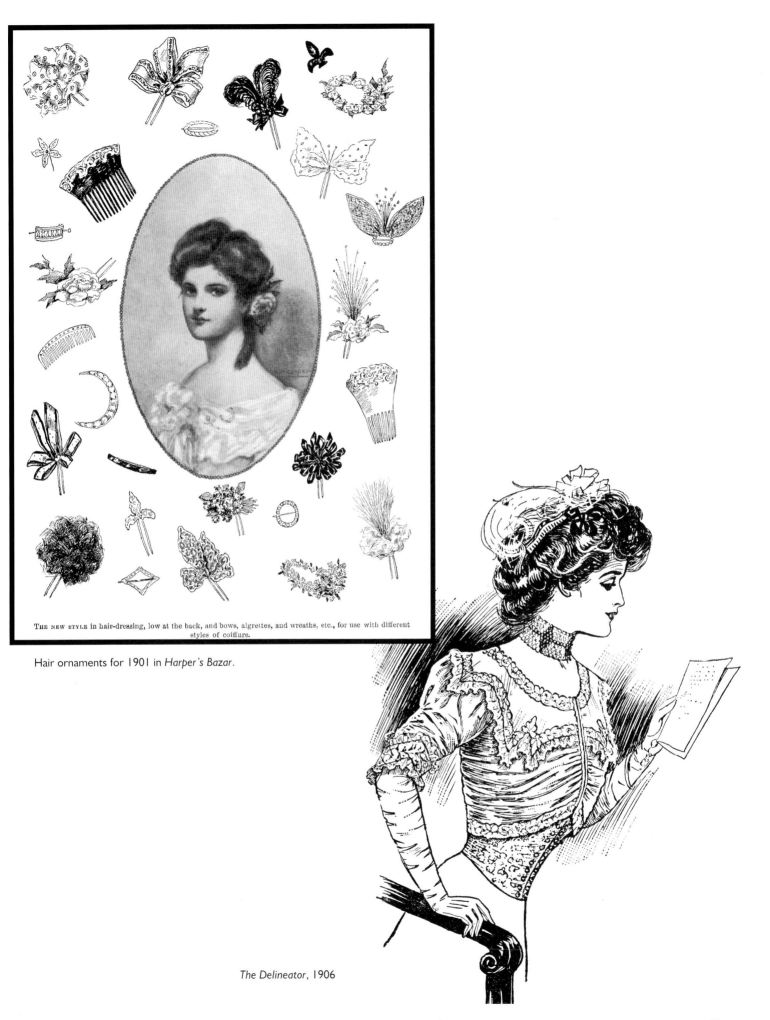

The NEW STYLE in hair-dressing, low at the back, and bows, aigrettes, and wreaths, etc., for use with different styles of coiffure.

Hair ornaments for 1901 in *Harper's Bazar*.

The Delineator, 1906

Good Taste and Bad Taste in Dressing the Hair

Drawings by Anna W. Speakman

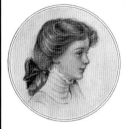

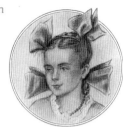

IF THERE is one thing more than another upon which a woman's looks depend it is the arrangement of her hair. The use of false hair is not to be despised, but, like everything else, the abuse comes from its overuse, and surely it has now reached the point where a halt should be called. Exaggeration in any form is always bad taste, but there is nothing in recent years which has become so pronounced as the craze today for overdressing the hair in the modern pillow-cushion style—virtually making a monument of one's head until all semblance of its natural size is lost. Perhaps it is the example of our steel-frame skyscrapers that has given a basis to the wonderful skyscraping structures built upon the average girl's head. As one man was heard to say to another the other day: "All that these things need to make them look like apartment-houses are windows and chimneys!" The Psyche knot and the puffs have reached such a pronounced and acute stage that one may call them the basis of the present malady in hairdressing.

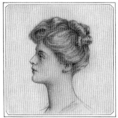

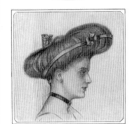

PERHAPS it would be well to say, as a fact and a matter of general interest, that hairdressing today, as it has been in the days of the past, is becoming to a woman only when it suits her own individual head. A general fashion of hairdressing is quite as absurd to imagine as a general fashion in food. To arrange the hair in the present preposterous styles is not only bad taste but it really has reached the point where it is the subject of caricature by the comic magazines. Hair to be properly dressed should, first of all, be well cared for and groomed daily, which means that it must be kept clean and frequently brushed; then it should be arranged to conform with the size and proportions of the head. To be sure, it is often necessary to use a certain amount of false hair, but this should always be used as moderately as possible, and so cleverly that, to the casual observer, it will seem to be a part of the real hair. It is unpardonable to pile on false hair at the sacrifice of the true lines and proportions of the human head, giving a top-heavy and overweighted decoration which deceives no one as to its artificial nature.

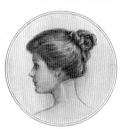

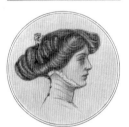

ON THE right side of this page the pictures show a few of the more exaggerated types of the present fashions in hairdressing, in contrast with the styles on the left, which are arranged to suit the different faces and hair. To begin with, the most misunderstood point in hairdressing today is in the arrangement of the pompadour: it is usually very exaggerated in its height and width, or it is so flattened down and tightly drawn back from the forehead as to give a hard, forced appearance to the face. It is well to remember that the hair should always soften and frame the face, and, if the word may be used, "gently" frame it. A hard, unbroken line around the face is most unbecoming to the average woman. A tight, rigid pompadour like the one above does not suggest human hair—it looks as if it were rolled over wood and painted. Such a pompadour is quite as distinct from the face and person as though it were a hat which could be changed and worn at different times and in various colors.

It should not by any means be understood that it is bad taste to wear puffs if they are worn in the right way and place. Look, for instance, at the girl on this page with a row of puffs in a straight, unbroken line directly across the front above the pretty, young forehead, set between her "iron-band" pompadour! Then, in contrast, notice the girl opposite, with the puffs worn low at the centre-back of the head, in a soft, beautiful arrangement that seems to be a natural coil from the medium-sized pompadour.

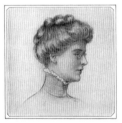

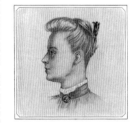

THEN there is the woman on the right who is growing old, and who, instead of trying to throw soft shadows and lines around her face, drags the hair back unmercifully at the sides and twists it into a flat little knot at the top; then she usually tops this off with a heavy, sculptured comb, when there is hardly hair enough to hold a small barrette! The contrast between this woman and the one on the left side is sufficiently clear to make further comment unnecessary.

Another type which is seen constantly is the middle-aged woman who wants to look young, and who tries to do it by making a bird's-nest of artificial hair and puffs on the top of her head, thrust out over an immense scoop pompadour waved in hard, unnatural lines. Compare this with the woman opposite, with her head of well-brushed hair arranged with a loose, natural pompadour which falls irregularly over her brow, and drawn gently back into a soft, big knot in the centre of her head.

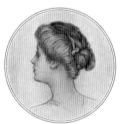

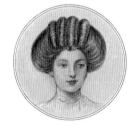

STILL another unfortunate type seen everywhere is the little child with tightly-combed and beribboned hair which looks like a miniature windmill—like the one at the right at the top of the page. With every breath of air you fear she will be suddenly whirled off her feet! Now, if there is one thing in the world that should be quite natural and simple in arrangement it is the hair of a young child, which needs only care to beautify it, as you can see by the young girl on the left. The present exaggerated ribbon fad among the children can be equaled only by the puff and pompadour fad among their mothers.

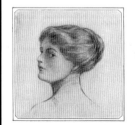

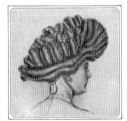

The Ladies' Home Journal, 1908

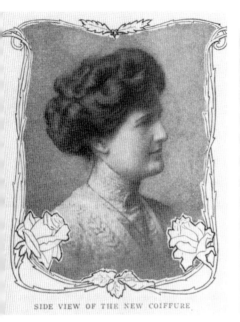

SIDE VIEW OF THE NEW COIFFURE

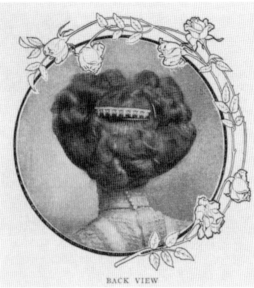

BACK VIEW

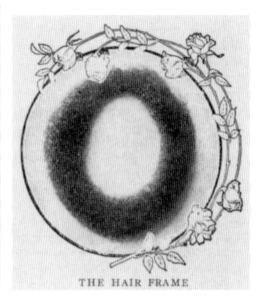

THE HAIR FRAME

McCall's Magazine, 1908

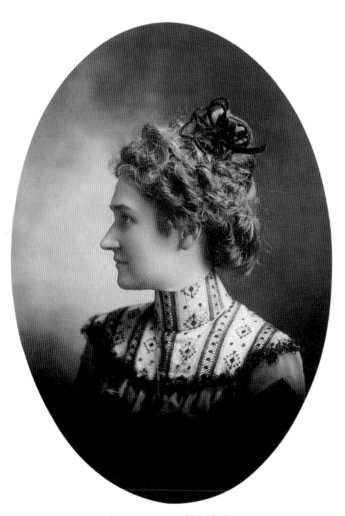

Chicago, Ill., c. 1906-1909

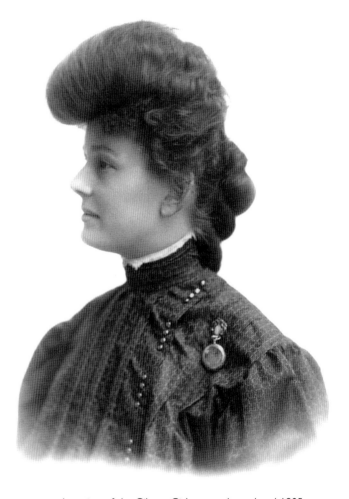

An exaggerated version of the Gibson Girl pompadour, dated 1905.

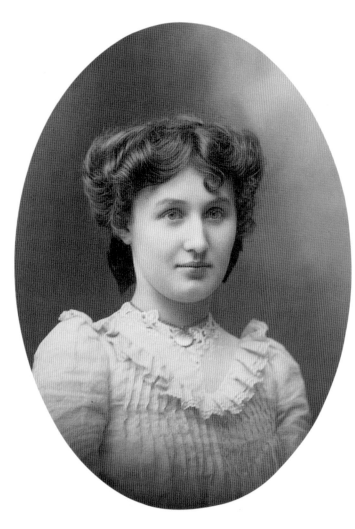

Landsborg, Kans.,
c.1906-1907

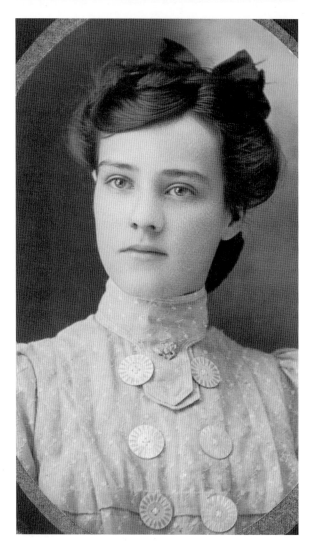

Leechburg, Pa.,
c.1904-1905

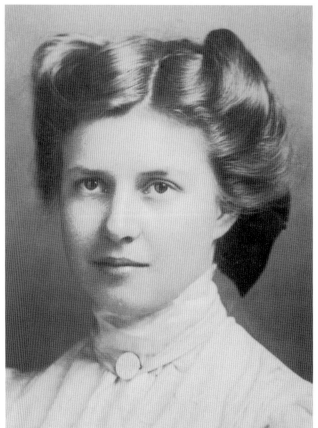

c.1905-1908

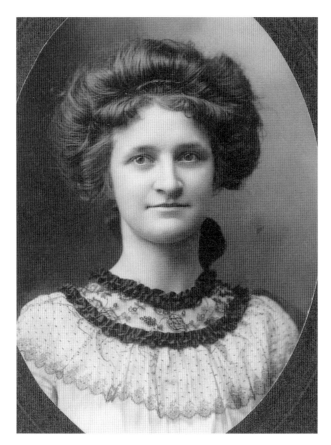

Landsborg, Kans., c.1906-1907

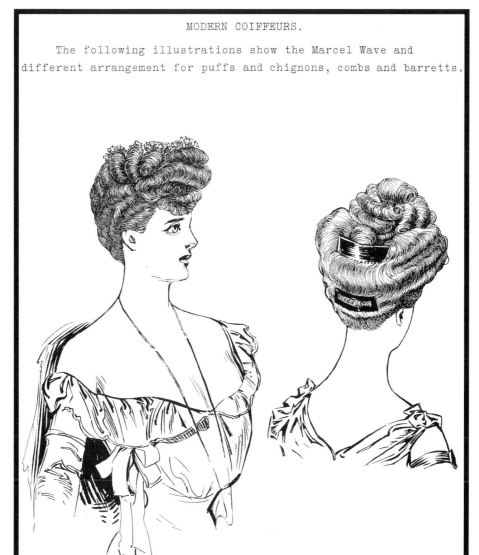

MODERN COIFFEURS.

The following illustrations show the Marcel Wave and different arrangement for puffs and chignons, combs and barretts.

From a hairdressing instructional booklet- the Marcel Wave of 1908.

1910-1920

The years from 1910 to 1920 were a time of fashion transition where few hard and fast rules existed. Many women still wore floor length skirts and stiff, chin-high collars while others adopted the shorter, flimsier modes that foreshadowed the relaxed dressing of the twenties. To say that any one style predominated in hairdressing would be wrong.

While the broadened pompadour was still favored for a time by the average woman, some looked to the past for their most glamorous coiffures. Long ringlets were seen, often in the company of water waves straight out of the 1870s. Full "psyche" puffs adorned the back hair in ornate arrangements reminiscent of the 1880s. Even the golden circlet of a Grecian band managed another revival. "Nothing is incorrect that recalls the head-dresses of the ancients," *McCall's* insisted in 1914.

Combs, hairpins and turbans graced the heads of those in vogue, along with what *McCall's* called "harnessings and trappings" of semi-precious stones, spangles, plumes and marabou. Ribbons of varying widths, and decorative bands became trendy with the younger woman, encircling loose layers of natural-looking curls and waves set the night before on large rollers.

"The woman who is always beautifully coifed for the street as well as for formal evening functions has graciously adopted the French twist," *The Ladies' Home Journal* happily announced in 1915. This newest incarnation sometimes rose almost beehive-like with a narrow band around the head as ornamentation or with a decorative pin at the side.

Hair fashion, it seemed, knew no limits, as modern beauty shops equipped with all the miracles that technology could provide sprang up in every small town. When *The News Record* of Apollo, Pennsylvania covered the opening of Mrs. Stewart's new beauty parlor in 1914, it noted that she provided "an electric hair dryer, vibrator, etc." and for one week would give ladies their choice of two treatments for fifty cents instead of the usual dollar.

It took a world war to swing the direction of hair fashion again. The young would emerge from it with their romantic illusions burned away and choose as their symbol of freedom and rebellion a style called simply "the bob."

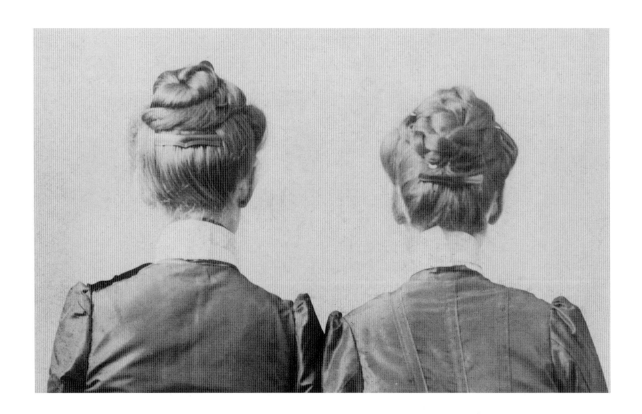

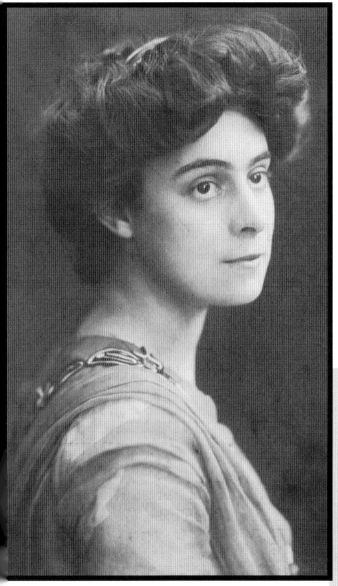

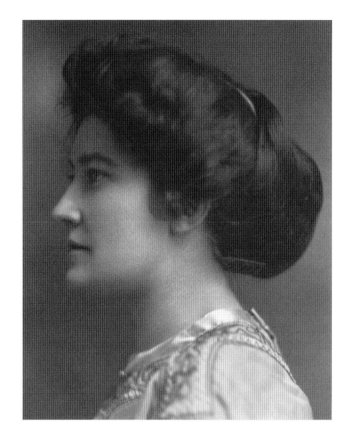

c.1910-1911

c.1910-1911

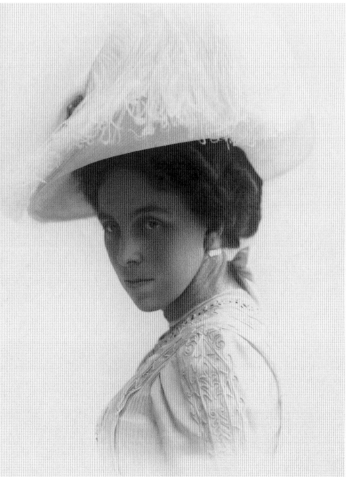

c.1910-1912

71

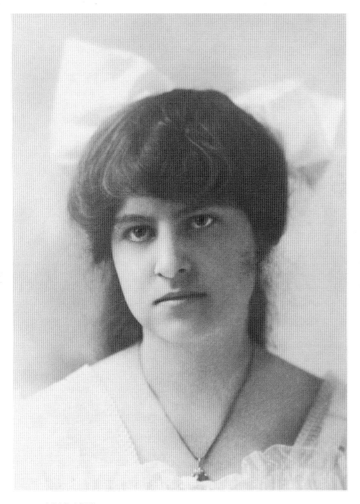

c.1910-1913

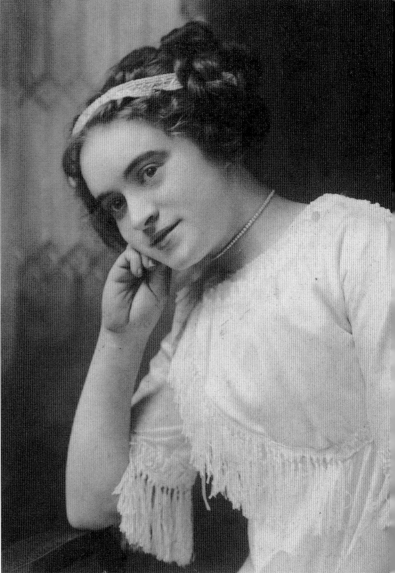

Turtlecreek, Pa., c.1911-1912

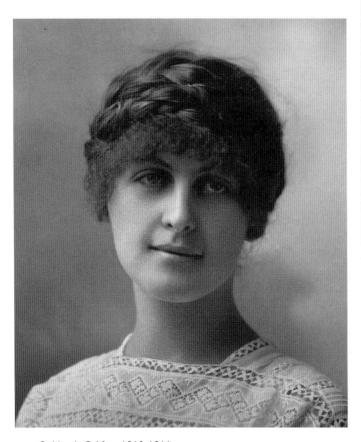

Oakland, Calif., c.1910-1911

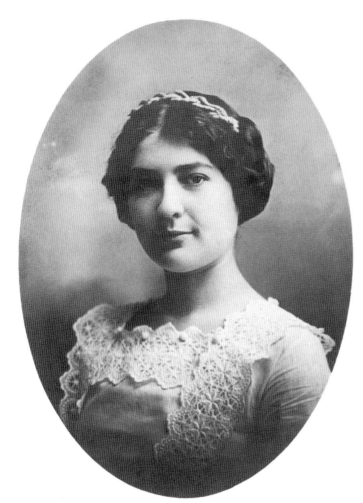

Monesson, Pa., c.1910-1911

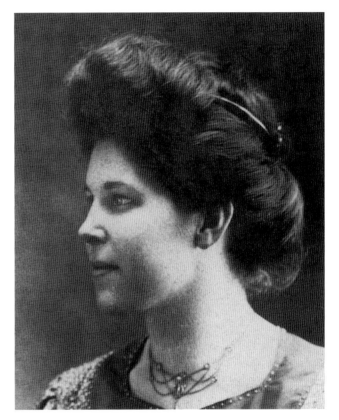

Parker, Pa., 1910-1913

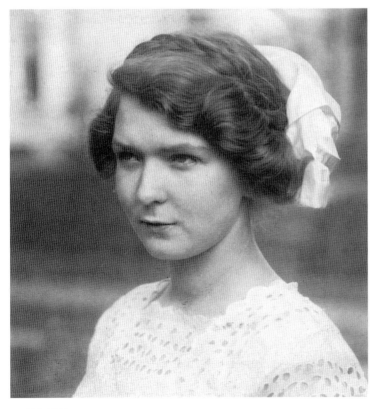

c.1910-1912

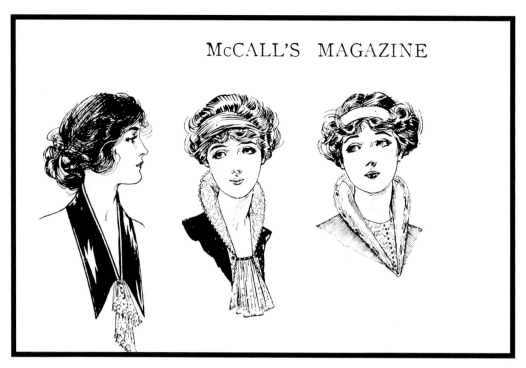

McCall's Magazine

McCall's Magazine, 1913

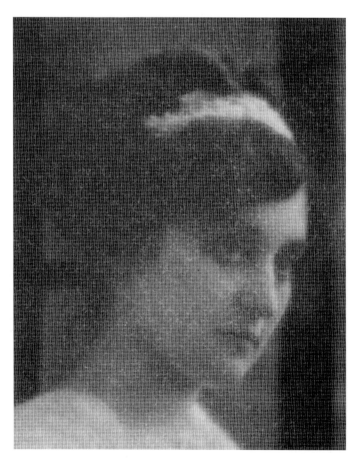

c.1912-1914

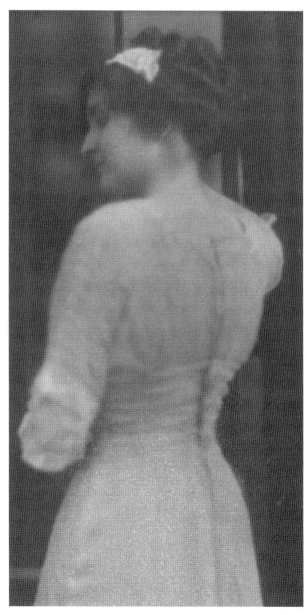

c.1912-1914

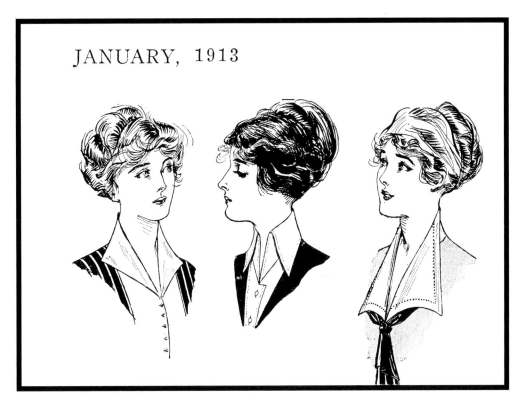

JANUARY, 1913

McCall's Magazine, 1913

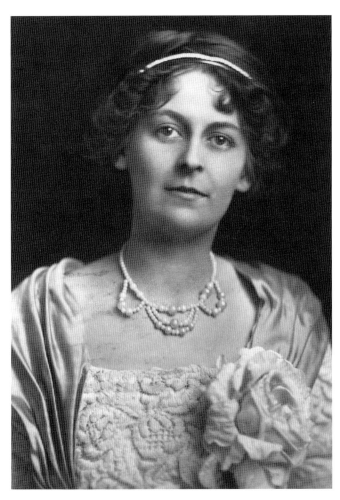

c.1913-1915

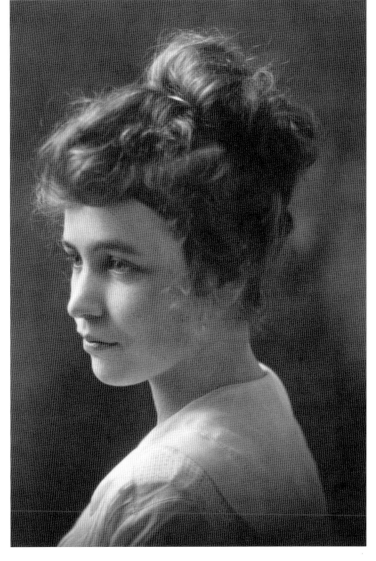

c.1915-1917

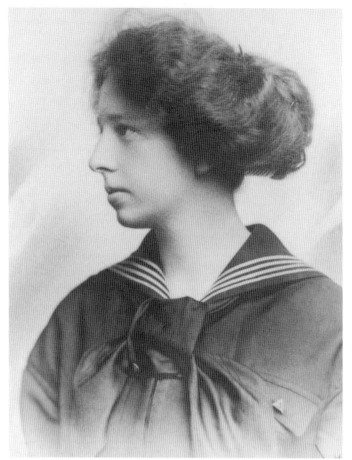

Waterville, Maine, dated 1912

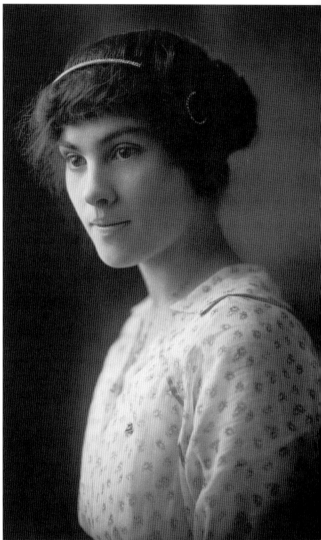

c.1912-1915

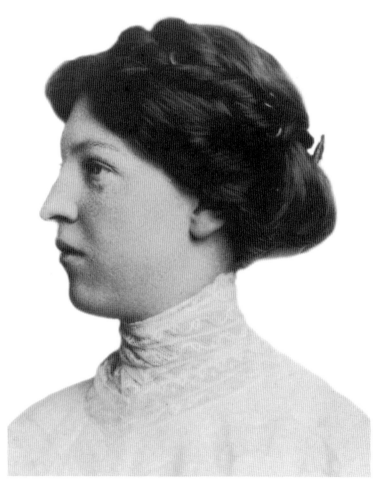

Waterville, Maine, dated 1912

The New Ways to Fix Your Hair

By Ida Cleve Van Auken: With Drawings by Anna May Cooper

UNDOUBTEDLY the gradual change in the styles of hats to the flatter crowns, with normal head size and fitting closely down on the top of the head, has been a strong influence for the varying arrangements in dressing the hair. To keep the lines of the hat low, so that it will fit down over the head, the hair must be worn smooth on the top of the head.

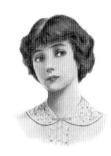

WHEN the crown of a hat is sufficiently deep the coils of hair, if worn low in the back, should be slipped under first and the hat then drawn down in front. If the weight of the hat rests on the coils it will push the back-hair arrangement out of place. After the hat is placed in position pull the hair out to form a soft fringe around the face.

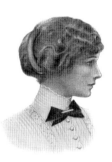

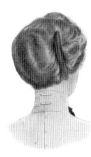

JUST above is shown the new invisible, twisted coiffure in a direct right-side view, while the back is pictured on the opposite side of the page. This coiffure is best adapted to smooth, loosely undulating locks, and is becoming to either a young girl or the more dignified matron.

A YOUNG girl with scant locks, medium forehead and round or slim face can wear her hair successfully as shown in the two upper illustrations in the center. The hair is parted in the middle, combed low over the forehead, and drawn together for the back arrangement.

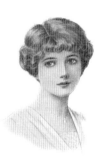

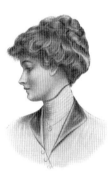

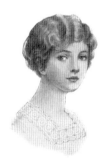

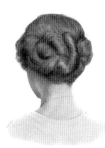

THE matron past her girlish youth prefers the distinctive height and graceful poise given by arranging the hair on the top of the head with a soft, loose pompadour around the face, as charmingly pictured in the becoming coiffure shown above and below, in two views. In the back the short ends may be caught in a bow barrette.

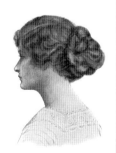

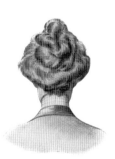

IN THE two illustrations above are shown an arrangement for luxuriant hair, suitable for a high forehead and a slim face, or for a fuller face. The narrow fringe shortens the height of the forehead.

More explicit directions for arranging the hair like these illustrations will be sent upon receipt of a stamped, addressed envelope.

ANOTHER charming coiffure is pictured in the two views above. The upper view shows the hair parted low on the left side and combed in loose waves toward the back. If the hair is not too wiry it may be curled naturally by dampening it and fastening it in loose waves with hairpins. Then it may be dried in the sun's rays, or with a warm towel.

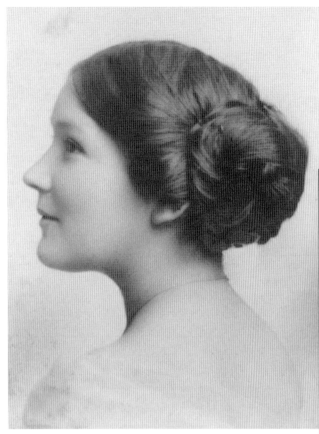

Waterville, Maine, dated 1913

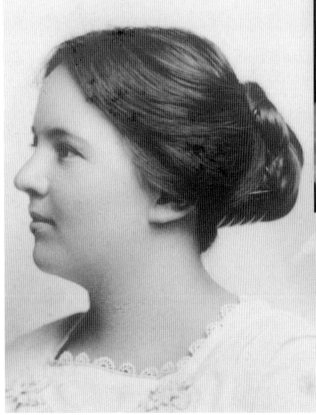

Waterville, Maine, dated 1914

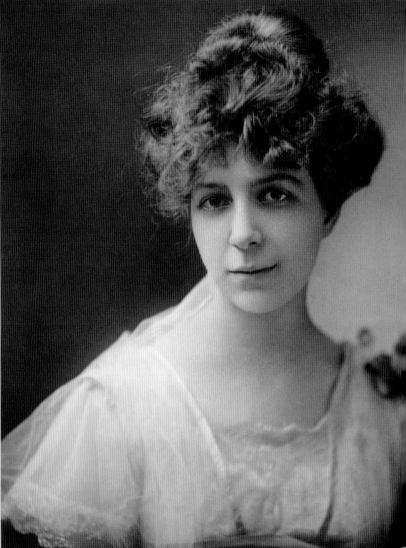

Boston, Mass., c.1914-1916

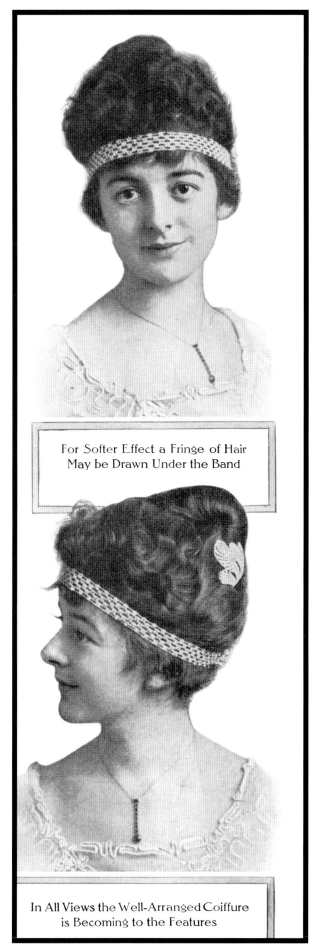

For Softer Effect a Fringe of Hair
May be Drawn Under the Band

In All Views the Well-Arranged Coiffure
is Becoming to the Features

The Ladies' Home Journal, 1915

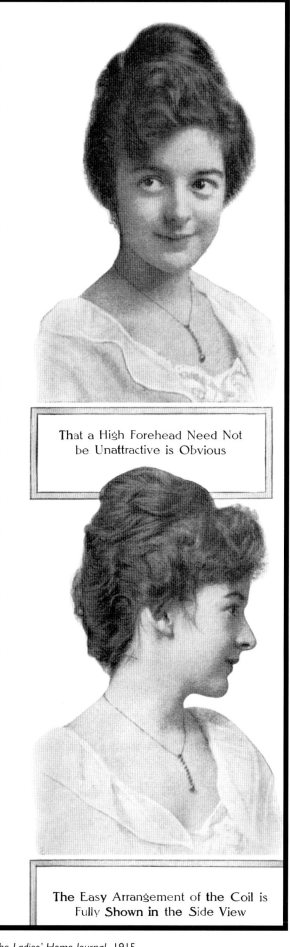

That a High Forehead Need Not
be Unattractive is Obvious

The Easy Arrangement of the Coil is
Fully **Shown in** the Side View

The Ladies' Home Journal, 1915

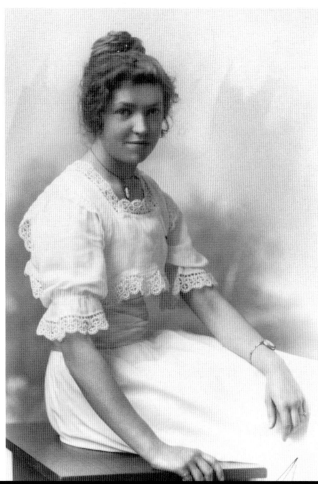

Ottumwa, Ind., dated 1915

The Ladies' Home Journal, 1915

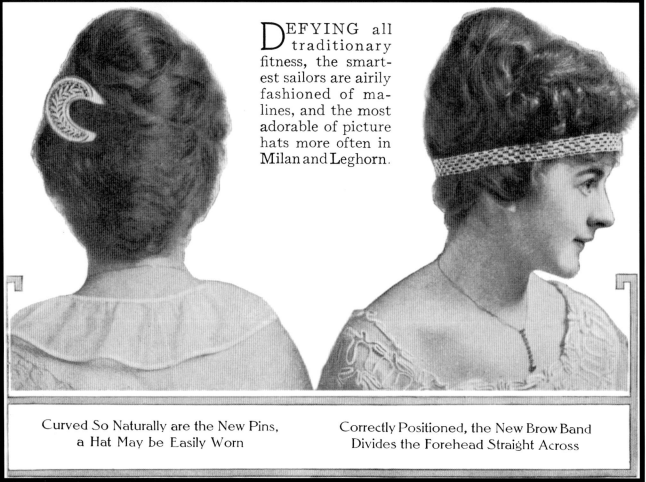

DEFYING all traditionary fitness, the smartest sailors are airily fashioned of malines, and the most adorable of picture hats more often in Milan and Leghorn.

Curved So Naturally are the New Pins,
a Hat May be Easily Worn

Correctly Positioned, the New Brow Band
Divides the Forehead Straight Across

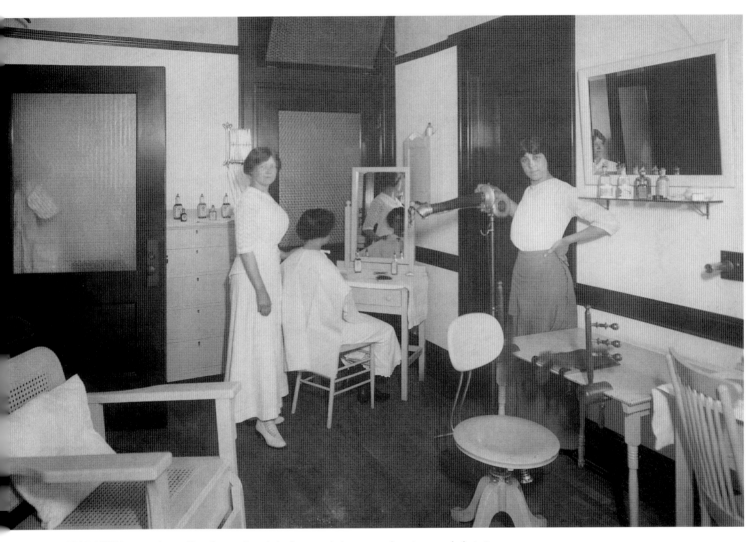

This c.1912-1915 beauty shop offered a modern hair dryer and also created custom made hairpieces.
(See one under construction at the right of the photograph.)

1920-1930

"Miss 1925—you notice has bobbed hair," said an advertisement for Ajax Bobbed-Hair Combs. "She bobbed it in 1918, let it grow long again in 1920—and then despite continued warnings from her elders bobbed it 'for keeps' in 1924." The bob was the signature style of the 1920s, forever associated with the flapper. Yearning for his elegant queens of the pompadour, Charles Dana Gibson dismissed the flapper as a "slimsy" sort of person. Many men agreed, resentful of young women who mimicked them in both appearance and manner.

"It is difficult to separate the lads from the lasses at the beaches this summer," *Men's Wear* complained in 1925. "The boys wear their hair longer than the girls, otherwise it would be almost impossible to separate the sexes." There were many versions of the bob. Some seemed permanently wind blown, some were softly curled, others were heavily marceled. Wide decorative bands were sometimes worn with the fuller arrangements.

The passion for curls had not died, however, and long sausage-like ringlets once more fell onto the shoulders and down the back. The chignon too was worn—Spanish style with a high comb. Those with bobbed hair who wanted a longer look for evening invested in a wig, called a "transformation" by the elite. The woman who retained her hair length experimented with a permanent wave.

The 1920s were a time of personal choices for women. Even color was more than ever before an option, thanks to improved new home dyes capable of tinting an entire head of hair in fifteen minutes. The vote was won, innocence was lost, screen stars set the fashion, and bobbed-hair flappers flaunted their daring in the face of old values that already seemed a world away.

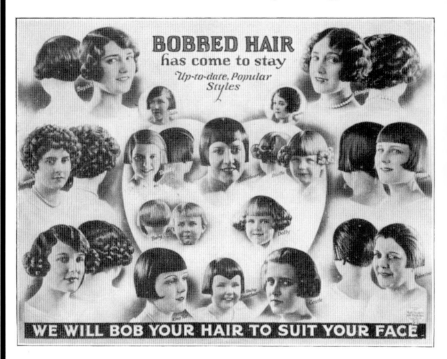

The above is a reproduction of our special chart No. S-1, which is made up in four sizes:

Photographic prints, size 17″ x 21″, mounted on a special finished cardboard supported by a double wing stand, price $1.50.

Photographic Prints, size 17 x 21, in colors, mounted on a special finished cardboard, supported by a double wing stand—Price $3.00.

Chart size, 14 x 18, printed on heavy cardboard with a glossy finish—Price $1.00. This sign is given with our Monthly Sign Service for Barber Shops and Beauty Parlors, as explained on page 35.

Chart size 22″ x 28″, printed with a glossy finish and mounted on a special heavy cardboard, supported with two substantial stands, price $1.50.

Ask your supply dealer or send your orders direct to Mah' Studios, 505 Fifth Avenue, New York City.

Beauty shop poster from 1924.

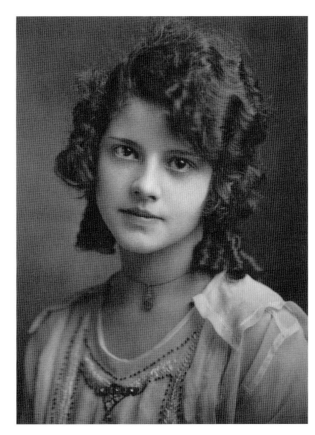

c.1922-1924

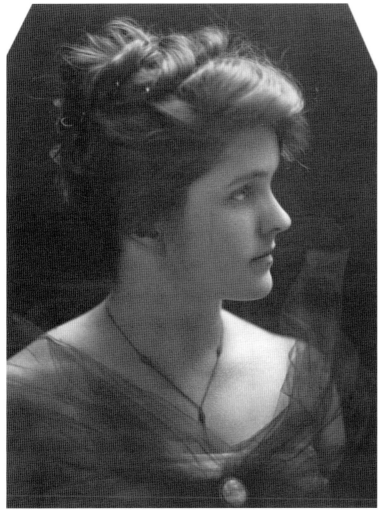

c.1922-1924

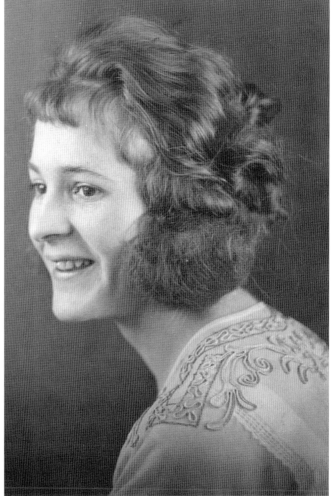

Dated 1921

83

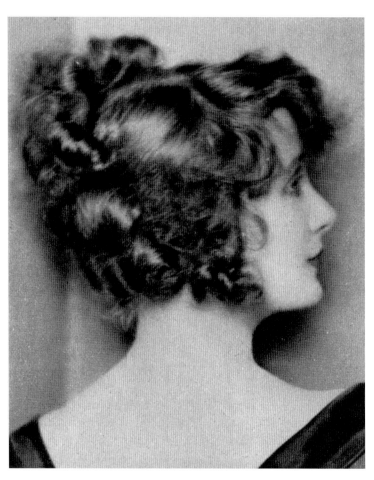

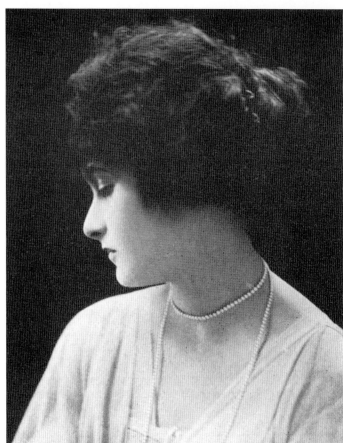

Screen star Billie Burke, 1923 photograph for *Beautiful Womanhood* magazine.

Beauty magazine, 1922.

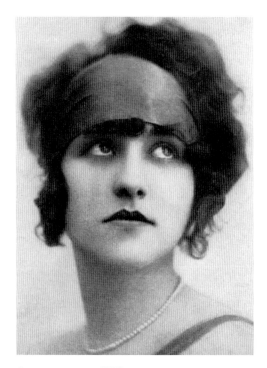

Beauty magazine, 1922

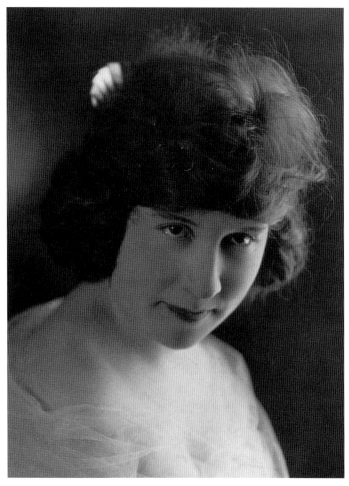

c.1920-1922

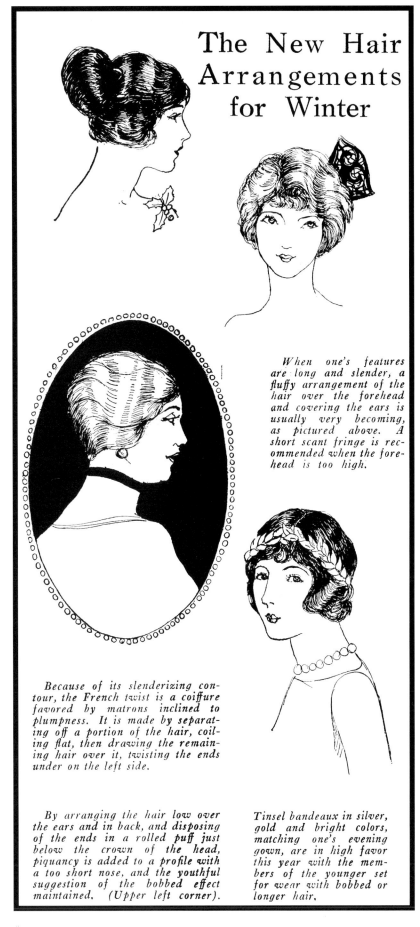

The New Hair Arrangements for Winter

When one's features are long and slender, a fluffy arrangement of the hair over the forehead and covering the ears is usually very becoming, as pictured above. A short scant fringe is recommended when the forehead is too high.

Because of its slenderizing contour, the French twist is a coiffure favored by matrons inclined to plumpness. It is made by separating off a portion of the hair, coiling flat, then drawing the remaining hair over it, twisting the ends under on the left side.

By arranging the hair low over the ears and in back, and disposing of the ends in a rolled puff just below the crown of the head, piquancy is added to a profile with a too short nose, and the youthful suggestion of the bobbed effect maintained. (Upper left corner).

Tinsel bandeaux in silver, gold and bright colors, matching one's evening gown, are in high favor this year with the members of the younger set for wear with bobbed or longer hair.

Today's Housewife, 1923.

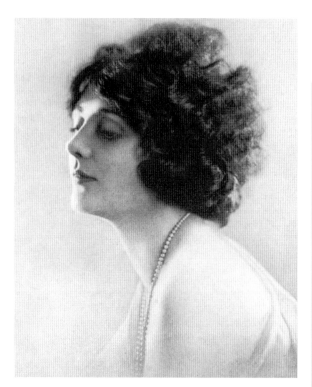

Beauty magazine, 1922

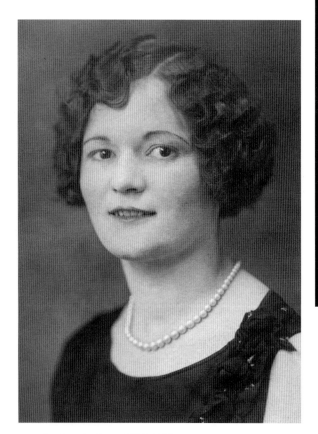

Pittsburgh, Pa., c.1929-1930

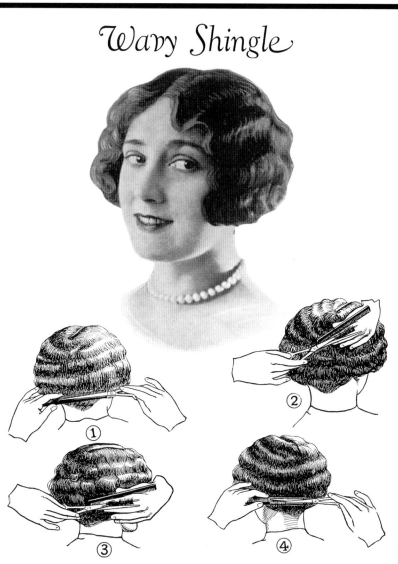

Wavy Shingle

This style of shingle is very becoming to women who have had their hair permanent-waved or desire to have it marcelled or permanent-waved after being cut. The method of cutting is as follows:

If the hair is already waved, commence cutting it at the back of the neck as shown in figure (1). Increase the length gradually to about five inches as you go upward by

Above and right:
The Tonsorial Artist, 1924

cutting the hair between your fingers, as shown in figure (2), and taper around the ears as shown in figure (3). Taper at the back of the head, working upward with shears and comb as shown in figure (4). In case of straight hair, which is to be marcelled or permanent-waved, cut the hair one inch below the ear lobe, so that after being marcelled or permanent-waved, the waves curl up to the position desired, creating a graceful appearance all around the head. Cut fuzzy hair from the neck with fine clippers or remove with hair remover.

When the bob is complete, it should look exactly like the central figure.

Natural Curly Shingle

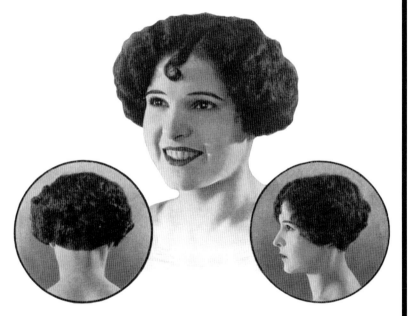

The natural curly shingle should be cut exactly as the Wavy shingle, only a trifle shorter, as shown in the above photographs. Instructions may be found on pages 10 and 11.

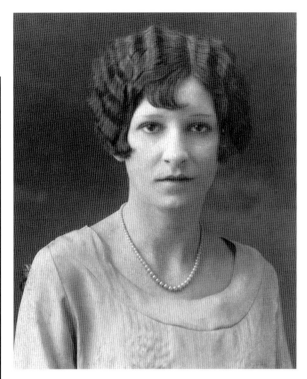

c.1929-1930

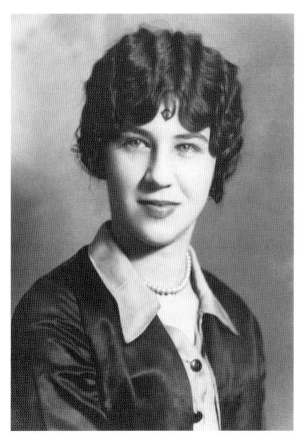

Apollo, Pa., dated 1929

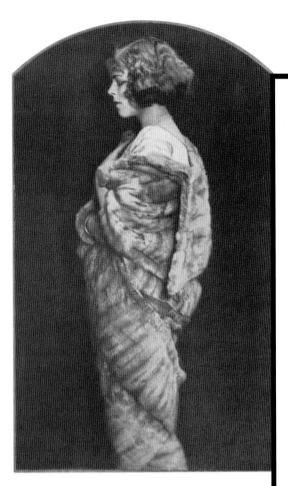

Beauty magazine, 1922

Senorita

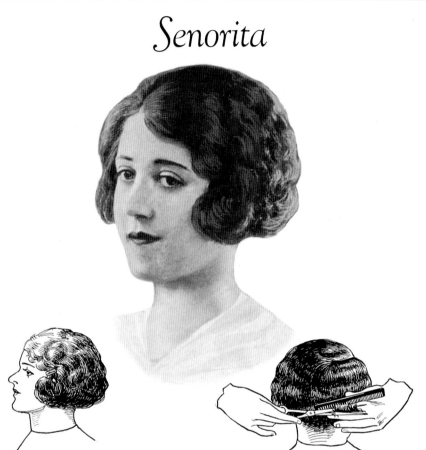

②   ①

This style is for women with naturally long, curly hair. It should be cut as follows:

FIRST:—Part the hair at the side, and brush down firmly all around. Start the hair line about one-half inch below the ear lobe, cut even all around, and taper the extreme ends gracefully by holding the hair between your fingers, as shown in figure (1). The hair may be pinned up at the side over the left eye with an invisible hair pin or barrette as shown in figure (2).

Remove hair from the neck if necessary, with fine sharp clippers or hair remover.

When the bob is finished, it should look exactly like the central figure.

The time required to complete this bob should not exceed fifteen (15) minutes.

Above and right:
The Tonsorial Artist, 1924

Lee Bob

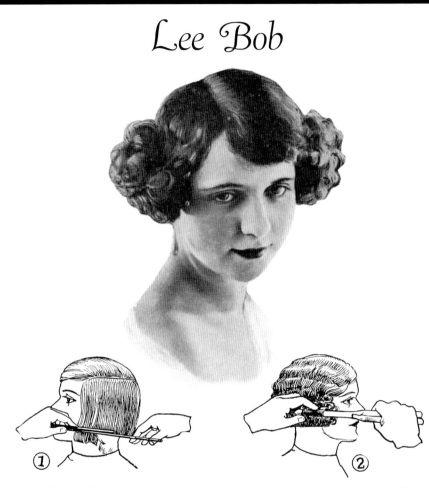

This style may be worn very becomingly by women who have natural wavy hair, or those who wish to have their hair curled after being cut.   It should be cut as follows:

FIRST:—Part the hair at the side, and brush down firmly all around.   Start the hair line about one-half inch below the ear lobe, cutting evenly all around as shown in figure (1).   Then taper the extreme ends by holding the hair between your fingers as shown in figure (1) on page 28.   The hair should be worn on the forehead with the dip toward the right eye, using an invisible hair pin to keep the hair in place.

For women with straight hair, desiring the Lee Bob, the same instructions should be followed, only the hair should be cut one-half an inch longer in order to obtain the desired effect.   Then curl all around with a curling iron as shown in figure (2).

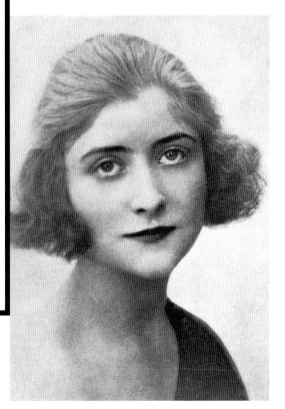

Beauty magazine, 1922

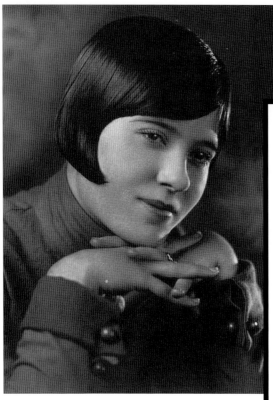

c.1924-1926

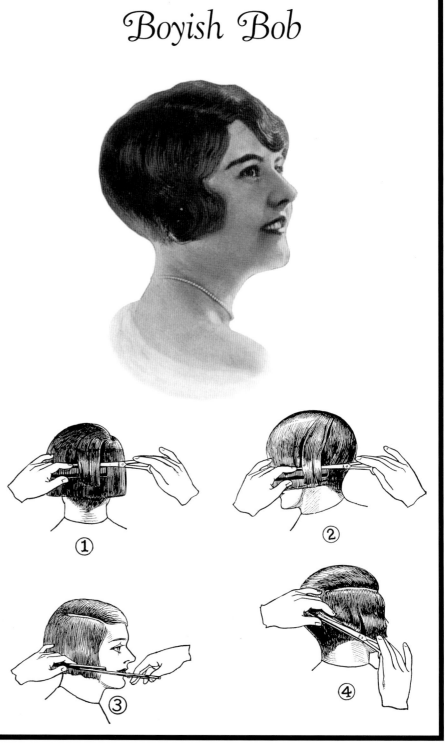

Boyish Bob

①

②

③

④

Above and right:
The Tonsorial Artist, 1924

slightly downward at each side towards the temple, there-by creating the effect shown in the central figure.

If the hair be thick or unruly, pomade or some standard hair preparation may be used to obtain the desired effect.

Remove hair from the neck up to where it has been cut, always using clippers or hair remover.

The time required to complete this bob should not exceed fifteen (15) minutes.

French Bob

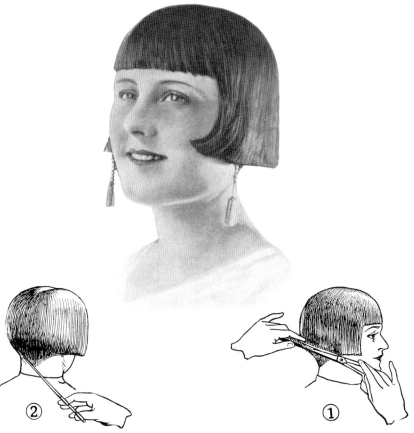

This is a Parisian style and should be bobbed as follows:

FIRST:—Part the hair in the middle and brush down firmly all around. Start your hair line right below the ear lobe. Shingle the back as you would in a boyish bob. Cut gracefully as you work upward to a point in line with

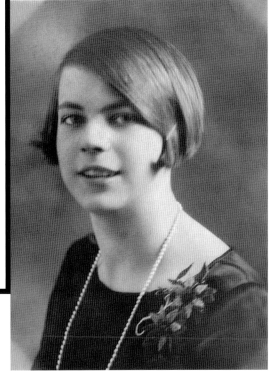

c.1924-1926

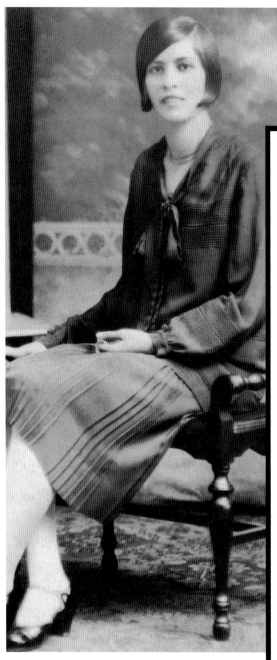

c. 1926-1927

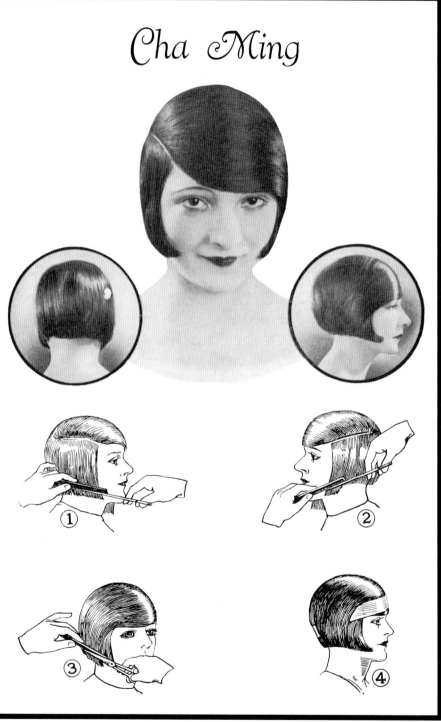

Cha Ming

Above and right:
The Tonsorial Artist, 1924

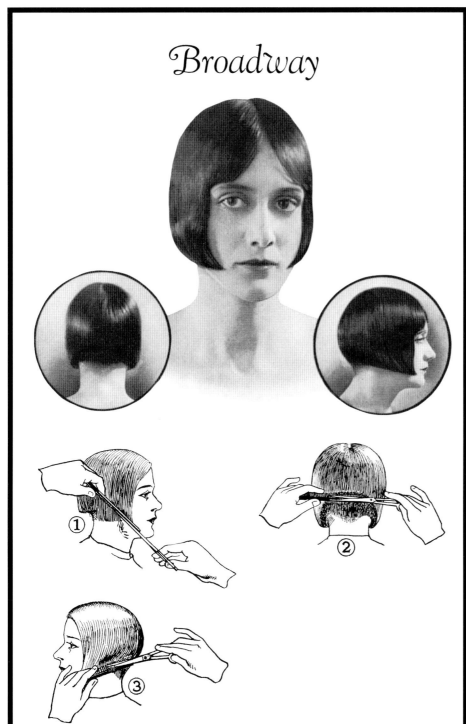

Broadway

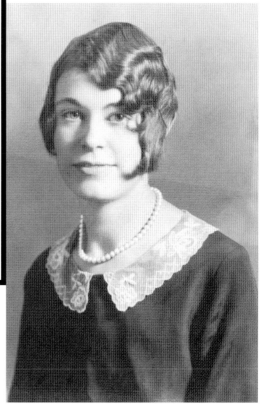

Apollo, Pa., dated 1925

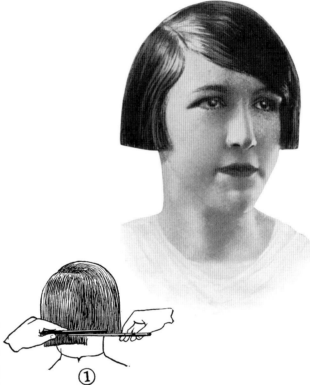

Vallie

① ②

This style is very becoming to young women with straight hair, but it may also be worn with a light wave whether natural or otherwise. It should be cut as follows:

FIRST:—Part the hair at the side and comb down carefully all around. Start the hair line slightly below the ear lobe, exercising care to form a perfect, straight line all around the head, by holding the shears and comb as shown in figure (1).

This style of hair bob should be worn slanting gracefully toward the right eye, using a barrette or invisible hairpin to hold the hair in the desired position.

Remove the hair from the neck with fine sharp clippers.

When the bob is finished, it should look exactly like the central figure.

The time required to complete this bob should not exceed fifteen (15) minutes.

Above and right:
The Tonsorial Artist, 1924

c.1926-1928

Dutch Bob

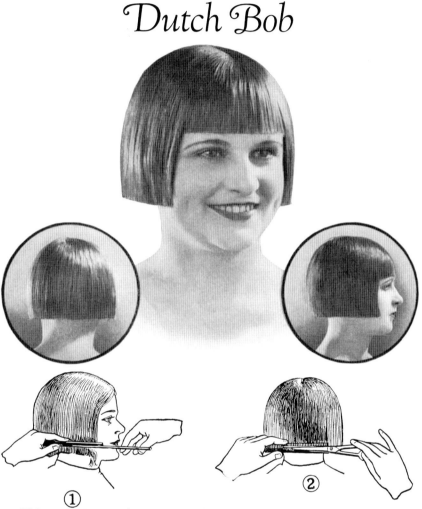

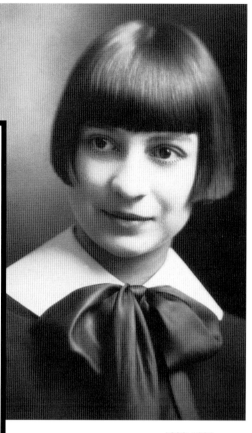

c.1929-1930

①   ②

This style is very becoming to blondes whose hair shows a tendency to curl at the ends toward the neck. This bob should be cut as follows:

FIRST:—Part the hair in the middle and brush down smoothly all around. Start your hair line one-half inch below the ear lobe, and keep a straight line all around the head as shown in figure (1). After you have obtained a perfect even line all around the head, if the hair hasn't a natural tendency to curl toward the neck, taper the extreme edges, working, with shears and comb as shown in figure (2), thus forming a club effect.

SECOND:—To form the bangs, brush the hair down on the forehead. Starting about one inch above the hair line, cut straight across from temple to temple a trifle above the eyebrows.

When this bob is complete it should look exactly like the central figure.

The time required to complete this bob should not exceed fifteen (15) minutes.

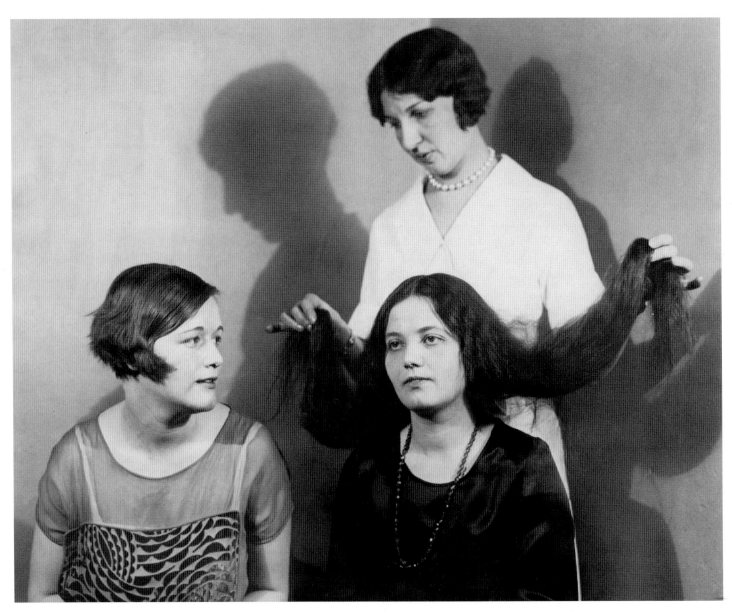

The "beauty doctors," at their 1927 convention, decreed bobbed hair passé. "Woman's crowning glory will be worn at its fullest length," they told the International Newsreel reporter—a prediction that would be a long time coming true. Short hair was comfortable and easy to care for, and women would continue to choose it in the future.

Chapter Three
Being Male

Men's Hair: Introduction

Only one rule held steady for men's styles from 1830 to 1930—the hair must be short. Wild West show stars might get away with shoulder length locks, along with artists, musicians and a general named Custer, but hair that descended very far below the ears was viewed with disdain on any other man. Parts moved reluctantly from side to center, the length and wave of hair at the forehead varied—small changes, which often escape all but the practiced eye. Only facial hair rescued men from hair fashion anonymity.

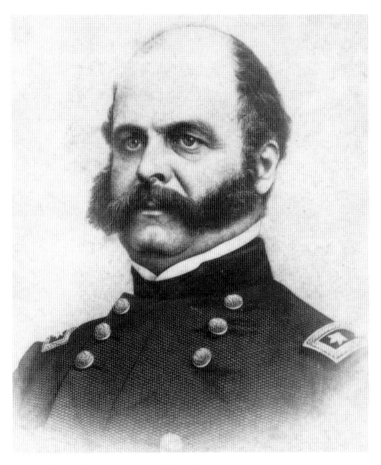

General Burnside turned side whiskers into sideburns during the Civil War.

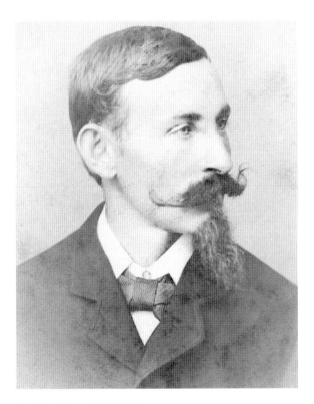

Franklin, Pa., c.1869-1870
The true T-beard or goatee formed a visual T from the front.

"We have almost as many accounts of the decline and restoration of beards as we have of the religion and politics which prevailed," *The Metropolitan* wrote in an 1872 review of past fashions. Until the mid 1800s there had been a general dislike of beards, though side whiskers and a fringe under the chin were tolerated. Mustaches had met with only cool approval. Acceptance for both came with the Civil War, when facial hair worn by admired military officers was immediately imitated.

Lee, Grant and others made a beard the mark of dignified manhood. Union general Ambrose Burnside merged his side whiskers and mustache in such a distinctive way that the name "sideburns" became attached to any side extension of facial hair. The most fashionable mustache of the 1860s was the T-beard or goatee. In its purest European form the stiffly waxed mustache combined with the elongated patch of beard to actually form a visual T. The American version was generally less stylized and far more dashing.

Mustaches appeared in seemingly endless variety from the 1870s through the early years of the twentieth century. The most prolific style was the handlebar—eternally associated with the "gay nineties." Its popularity ended abruptly, however, when Kaiser Wilhelm sported his meticulously waxed adaptation while dragging the world into war.

America's passion for well-manicured facial hair filled the masculine dressing table with specialized tools: mustache combs and brushes, mustache wax, a shaving kit containing as many as seven different razors, along with soaps, scissors, curlers and dyes. Many avoided the clutter with a daily trip to the barber.

During the mustache craze the barber shop became a male sanctuary of near sacred proportion—a place of polished mirrors, shiny porcelain, gleaming chrome, and racks of personalized shaving mugs and brushes for regular customers who hoped to avoid the contamination of "barber's itch." The 1889 editors of *The Family Herald* found it all too precious. "Barbers are becoming absorbed into tonsorial professors, artists in hair, coiffeurs, and possibly half a dozen other imposing styles and qualifications," they complained.

What critics failed to realize was that the modern barber shop fulfilled a real and practical need. It was there that friends were met, contacts made, news shared, and politics argued. And it was there that a man could reaffirm his maleness in a world increasingly intruded on by women.

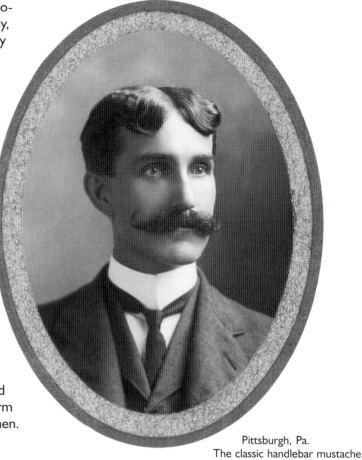

Pittsburgh, Pa.
The classic handlebar mustache of the "Gay Nineties."

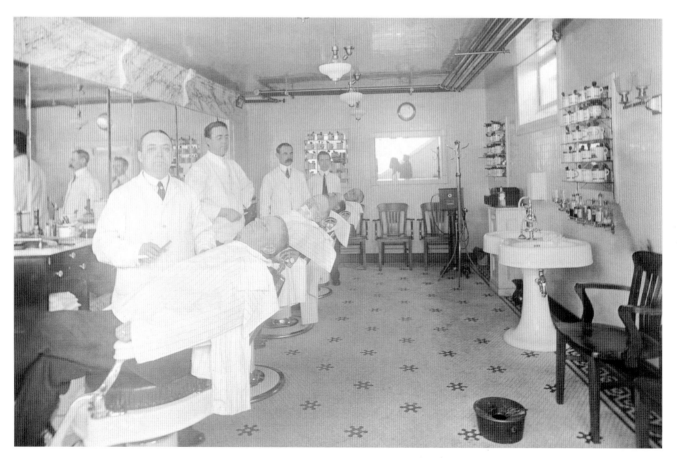

1830-1880

From 1830 to 1850 men wore their hair loosely waved over the forehead, slightly long and wide about the ears, often with an upward curl at the ends. The part was to the side, as it would continue to be until the 1880s. Side whiskers were common, as was a fringe beard. The gentleman of fashion was elegantly genteel to the point of femininity. In her book *Historic Dress In America*, Elisabeth McClellan quoted a poetic expression of disgust from the period: "They've made him a dandy; / A thing, you know, whisker'd, great-coated and lac'd."

By 1850 a change was evident. Hair was shorter and well greased with macassar oil, to the horror of women who covered the backs of their chairs with fussy anti-macassars in response. In 1854 *Harper's Monthly* named "the beard movement" the great social revolution of the age. By the 1860s both beards and mustaches were common.

Facial hair remained widespread through the Civil War years into the 1870s. Photographs of the time show that men were coaxing a graceful wave down onto their foreheads as well. For those whose hair was obstinately uncooperative, there were plenty of other options. "It is true that at the present time the greatest latitude is allowed in the matter," *The Metropolitan* assured them in 1872. "Men wear their hair and beards as they please."

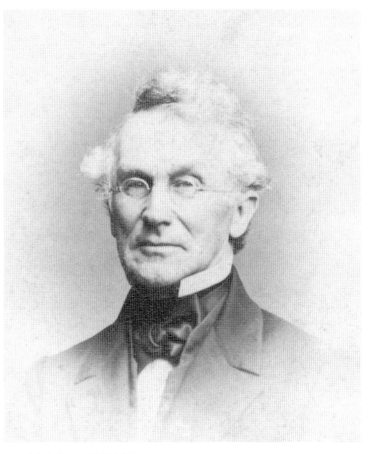

New York City, c.1858-1859

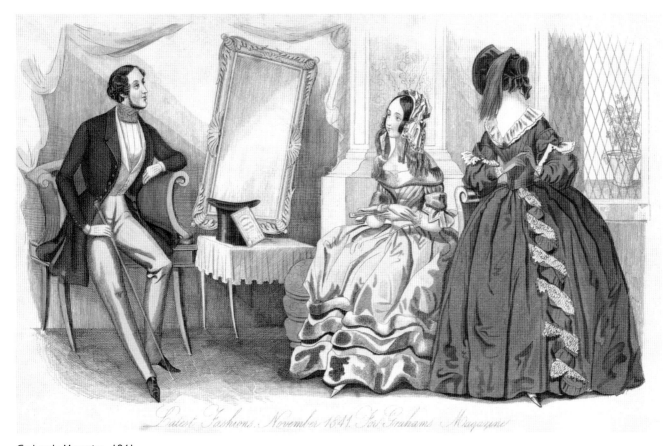

Graham's Magazine, 1841
"They've made him a dandy...."

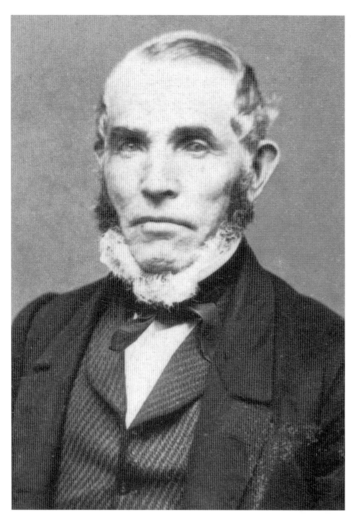

Syracuse, N.Y., c.1859-1860

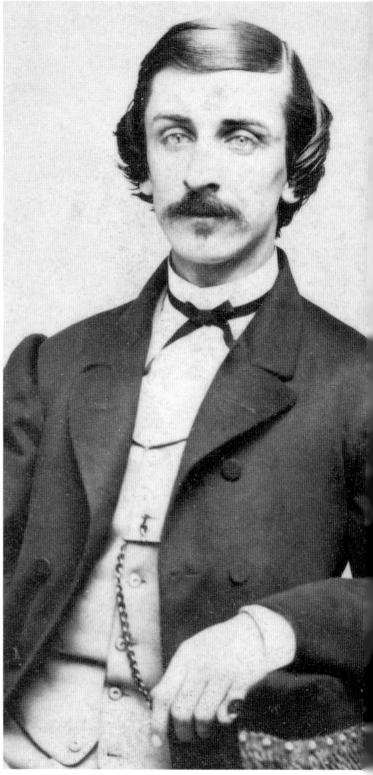

San Francisco, Calif., dated 1861

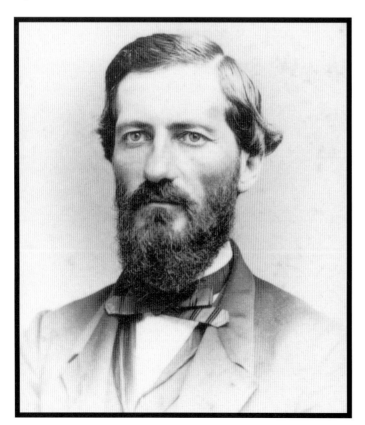

Philadelphia, Pa., dated 1863

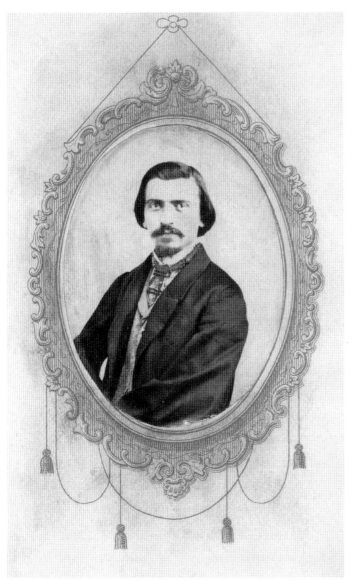

Ohio, c.1863-1865

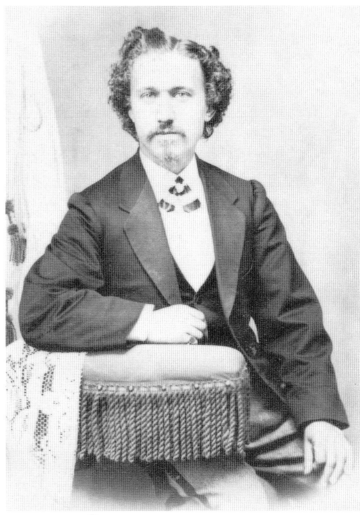

Pleasantville, Pa., c.1863-1864

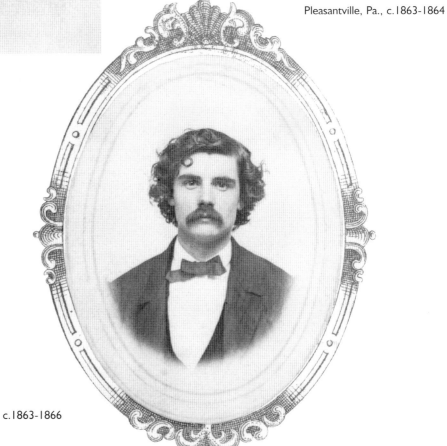

c.1863-1866

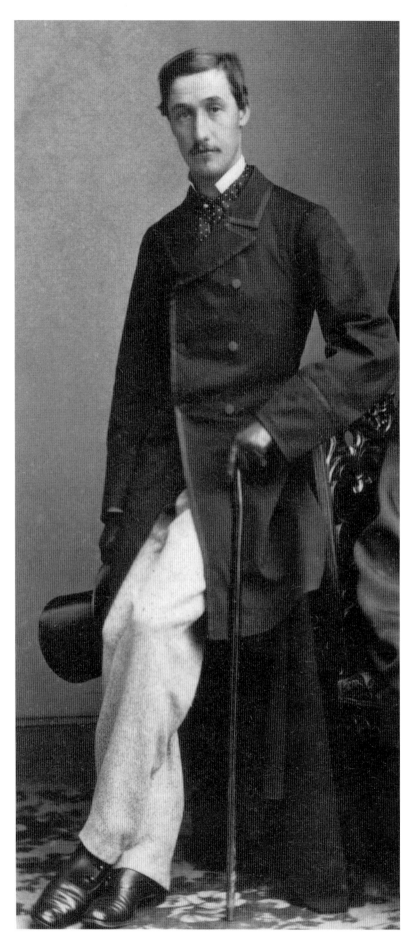

New York City man of fashion, 1863.

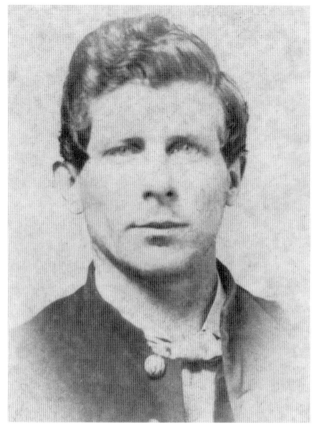

Company E 45th regiment Pa volunteers

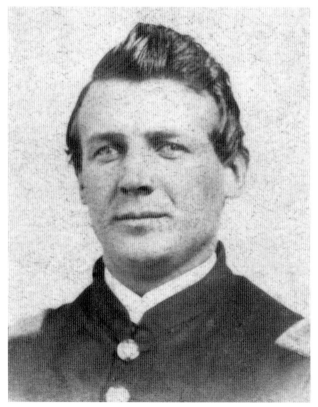

Washington, D.C.

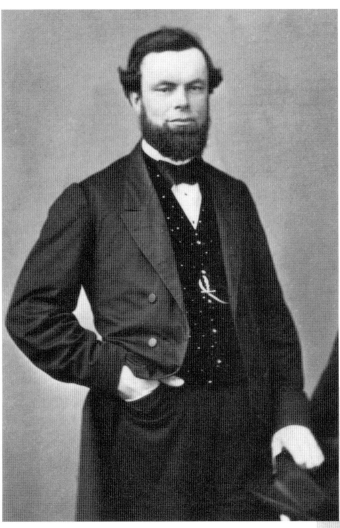

New York City, c.1864-1865

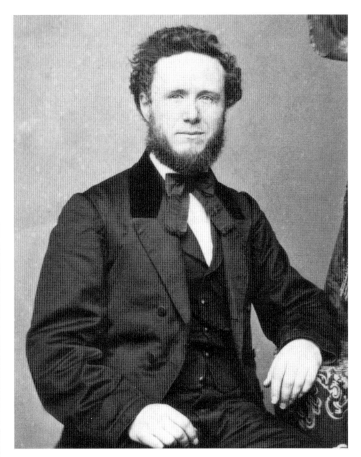

Philadelphia, Pa., c. 1865-1866

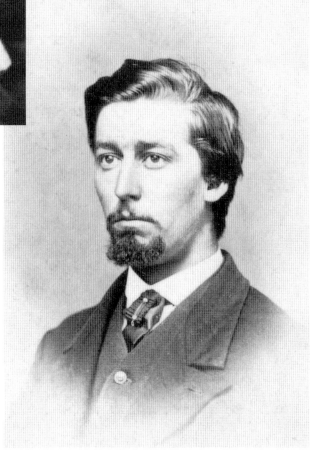

Peoria, Ill., c.1864-1866

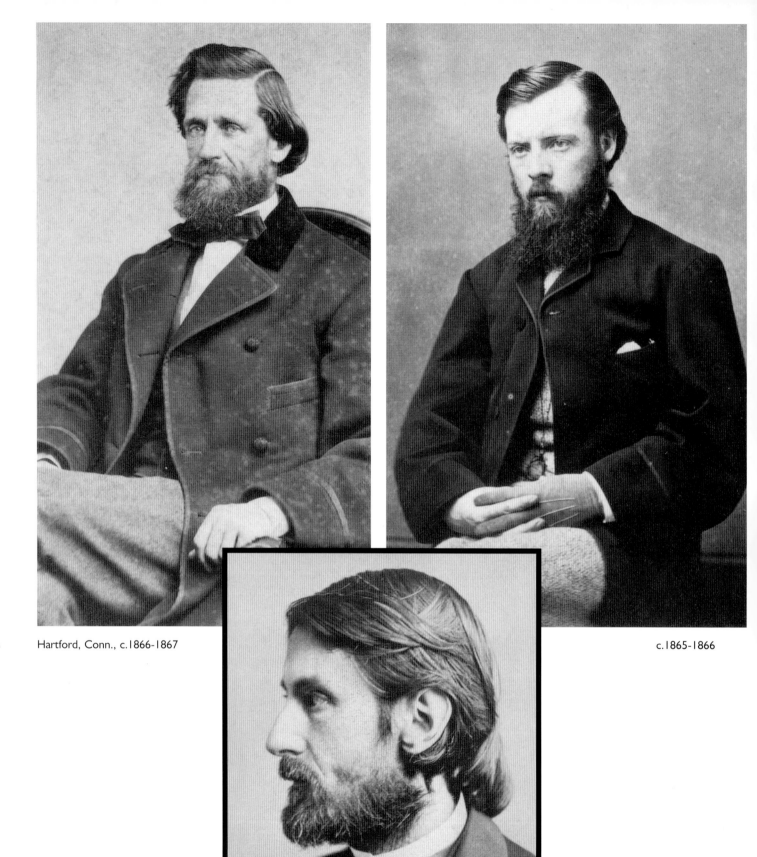

Hartford, Conn., c.1866-1867

c.1865-1866

c.1866-1868

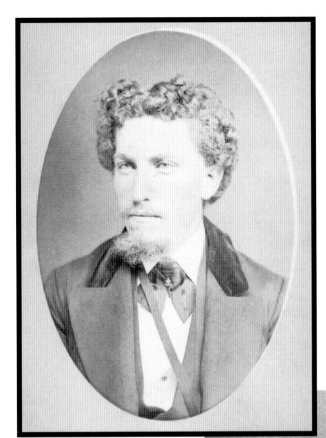

Reading, Pa., c.1868-1870

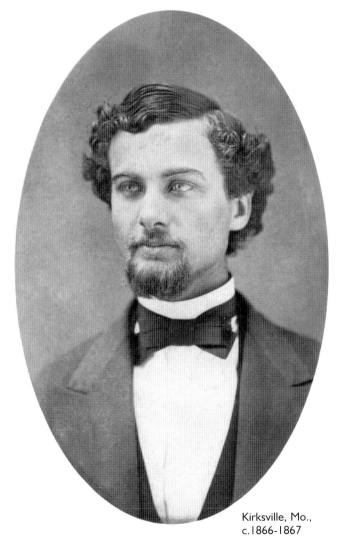

Kirksville, Mo.,
c.1866-1867

Ithaca, N.Y., c.1868-1870

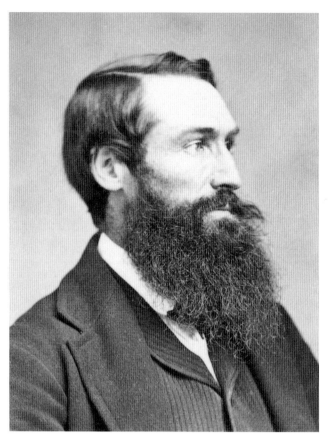

Montpelier, Vt., c.1866-1868

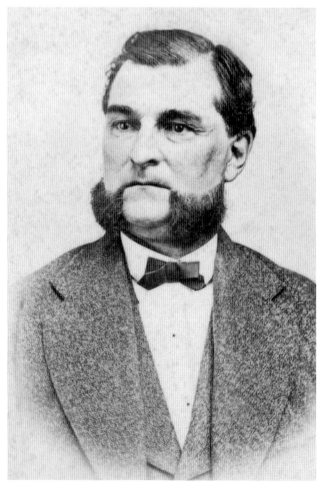

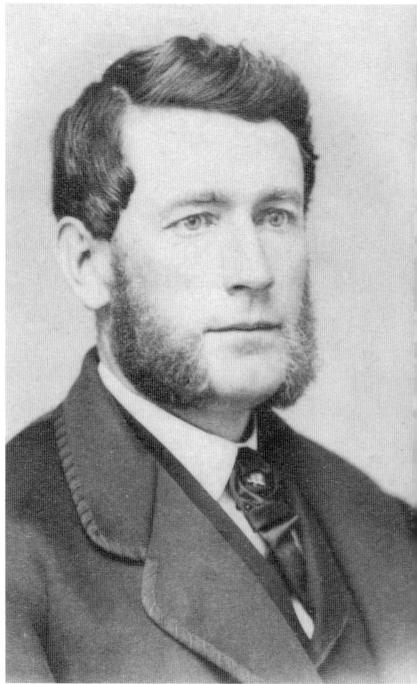

Waverly, N.Y., c.1868-1870

c.1868-1870

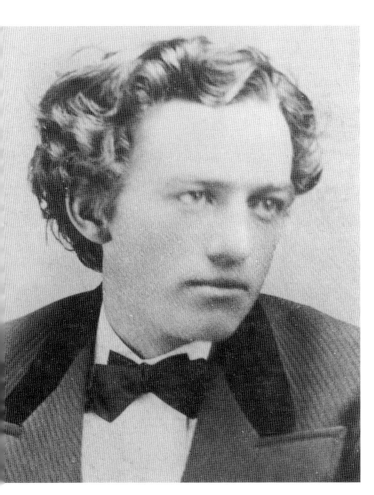

Greenville, Pa., c.1869-1870

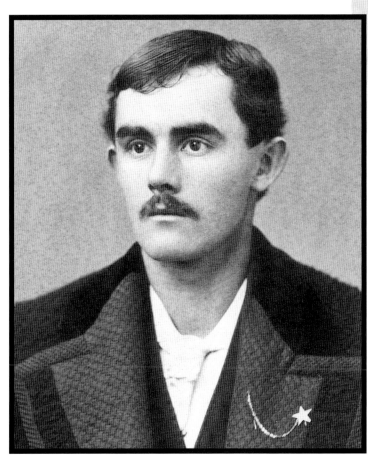

Urbana, Ohio, c.1870-1874

Washburn, Ill., c.1869-1870

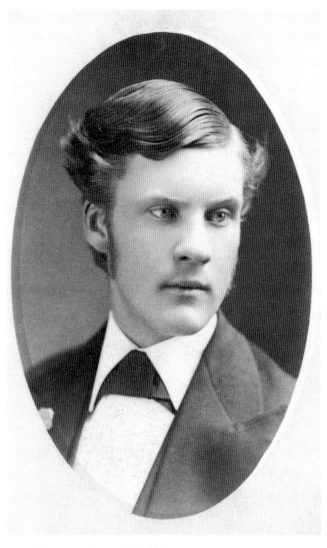

Delaware, Ohio, c.1870-1871

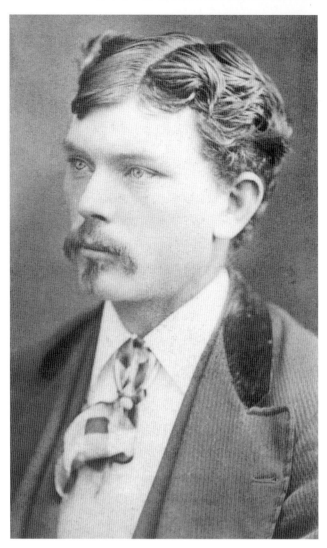

Chicago, Ill., c.1871-1873

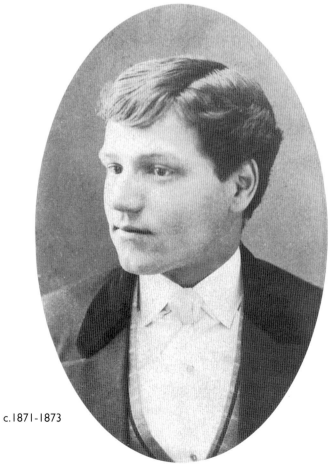

c.1871-1873

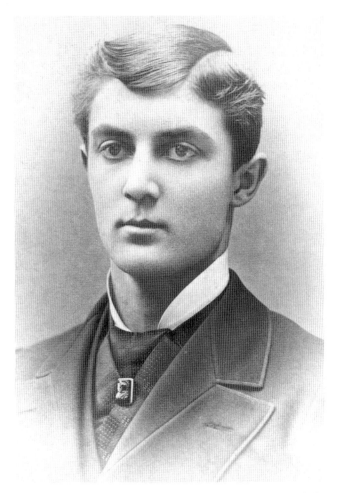

Titusville, Pa., c.1877-1878

Titusville, Pa.,
c.1874-1876

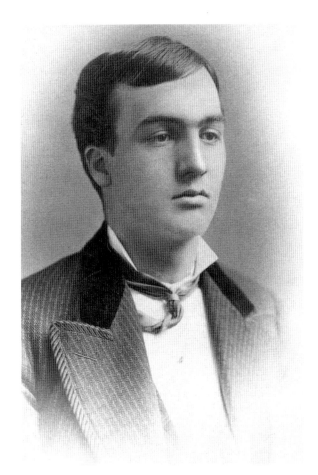

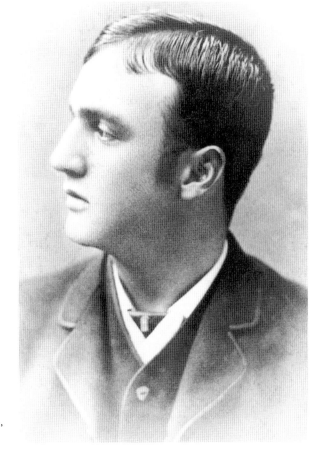

Titusville, Pa.,
c.1877-1878

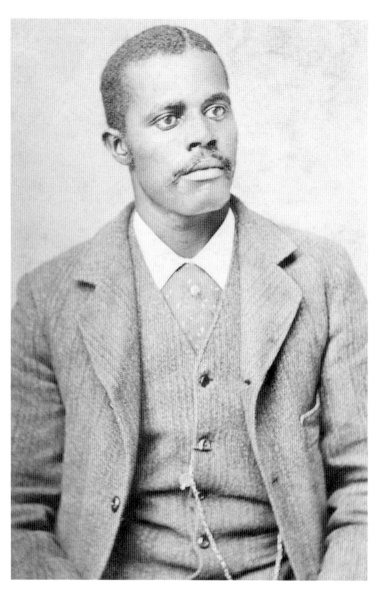

Norfolk, Va., c.1877-1879

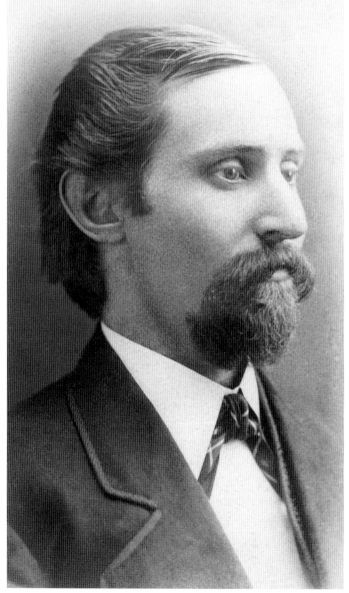

Chicago, Ill., c.1877-1879

1880-1900

In England, parts moved to the center. Americans seemed reluctant to adopt what had always been considered a feminine affectation, leading most men to hold steadfastly to the masculine tradition of the side part. The artistic swoop of wave over the forehead disappeared as hair was cut shorter and conservatism became the fashion rule for the head. The face was another matter.

Older men wore neatly trimmed beards and side whiskers, while younger men began sprouting amazing mustaches. It was a trend that grew through the 1880s until probably half of the males on any given street in America wore some version of the mustache, and virtually no public official went barefaced. As the century neared its end, however, the clean-shaven look was being adopted by the stylish young men who now set the fashion pace.

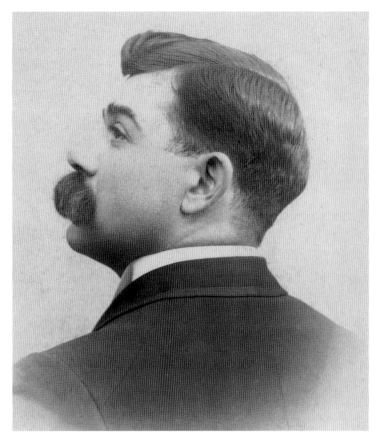

The man of the 1890s.

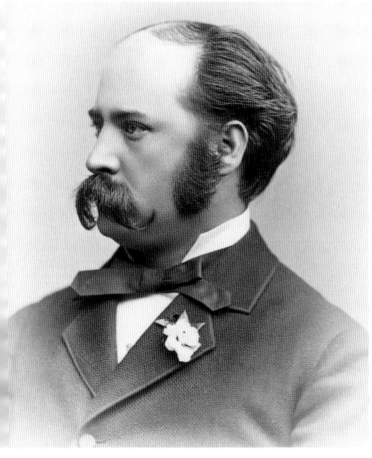

San Francisco, dated 1880

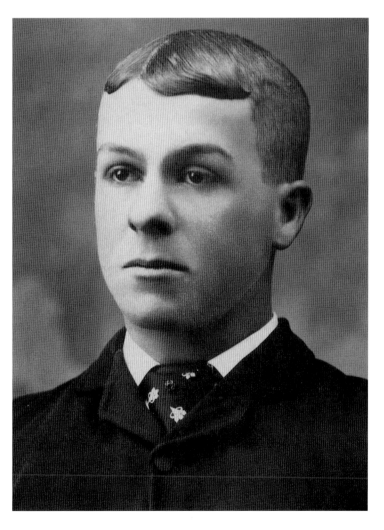

Battle Creek, Mich., c.1880-1882

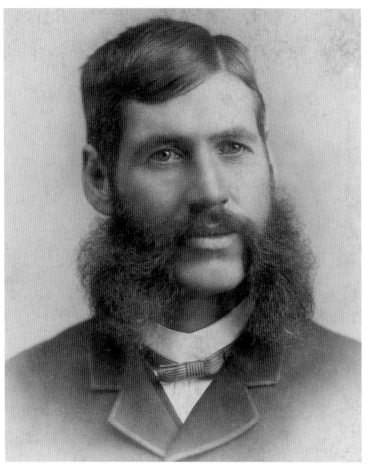

Bradford, Pa., c. 1880-1881

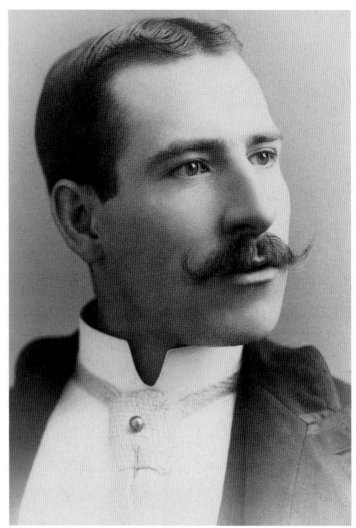

Albany, N.Y., dated 1888

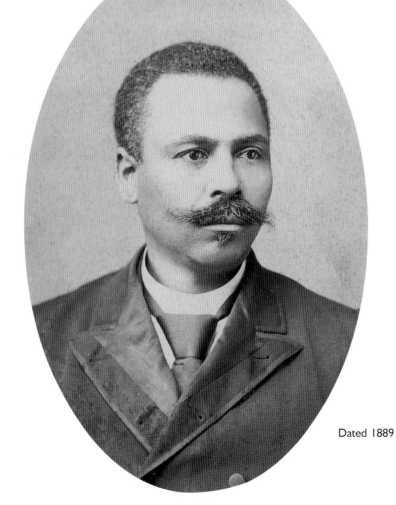

Dated 1889

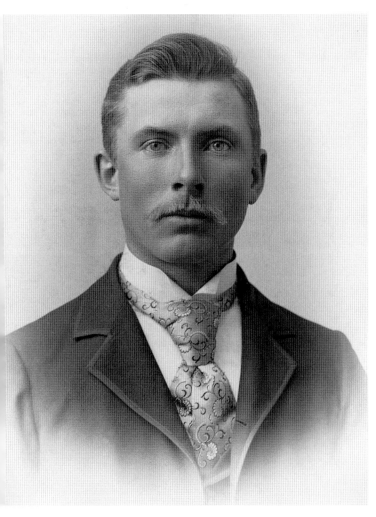

Carey, Ohio, c.1891-1894

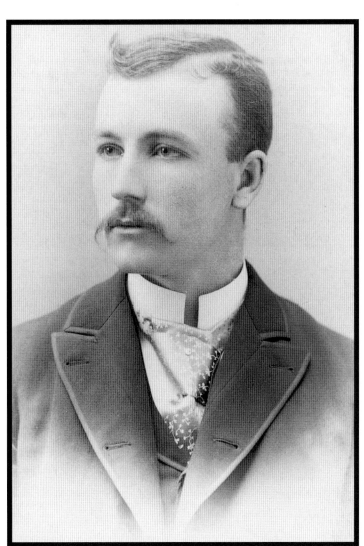

Hamilton, N.Y., c.1889-1890

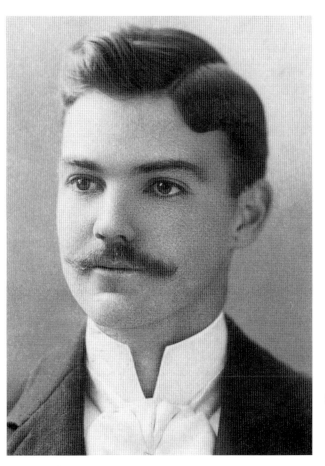

Boston, Mass., dated 1892

113

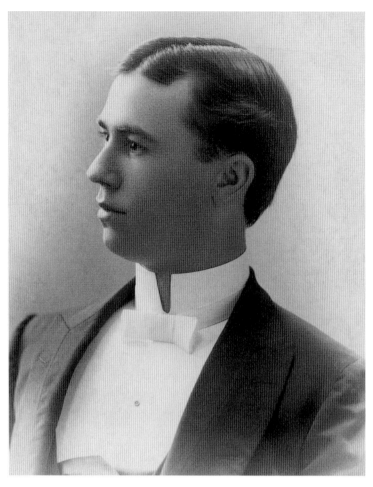

Ann Arbor, Mich., dated 1893

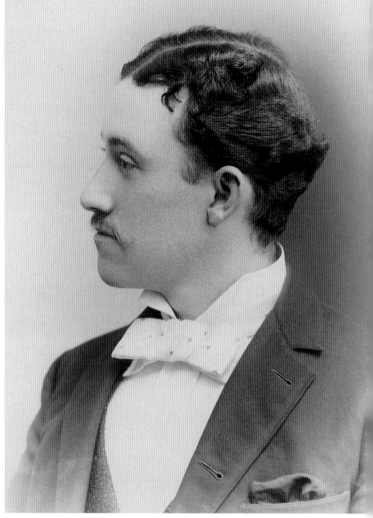

Newark, Ohio, dated 1892

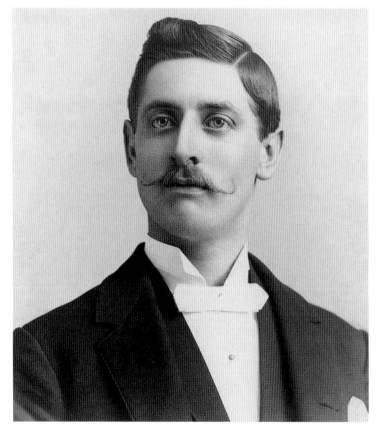

Zelienople, Pa., c. 1893-1894

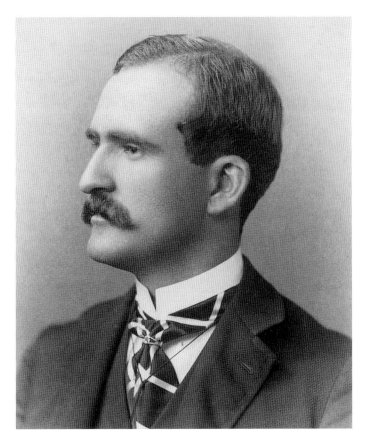

1900-1930

The turn-of-the-century man who stood proudly stroking his waxed handlebar mustache looked quaintly out of touch by 1910. The clean-faced new man, on the other hand, appeared completely comfortable in his modern era of automobiles, flying machines, and moving pictures. He was less prepared for modern warfare, unfortunately. He emerged from its horrors with shattered illusions and a determination to meet the future on its own terms.

"The clothier today judges his customer by his adjectives and his haircut rather than the class of merchandise in which he is interested," *Men's Wear* reported in 1923. Beards were still seen from time to time on the faces of the scholarly, but the mustache craze was dead. The emphasis had shifted to the hair.

"Attention is now called to the preparations that implant a patent leather finish to the hair and, while creating a halo not unlike Rudolph Valentino's, likewise impress the blessed damsels tremendously," *Men's Wear* wrote. The "preparations" that brought a man's hair to stylish perfection were basically the same as those employed by the thoroughly modern woman. By 1930 the man's world had lost its exclusivity.

Baltimore, Md., c.1895-1898

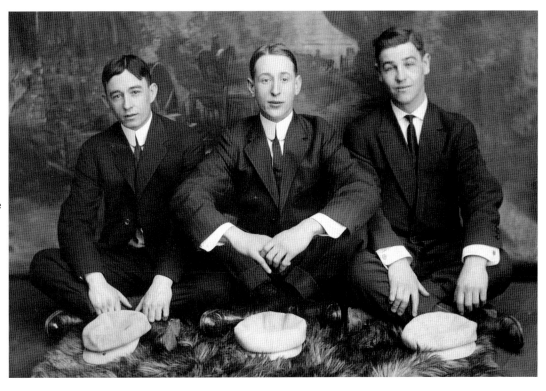

Three men of the modern world, c.1907-1910.

Both sexes used the same pomades and brilliantines, both shared the marceling iron and permanent wave, and both sported nearly the same bob. Even the barbershop was no longer sacred. Women now brazenly invaded that inner sanctum of male exclusivity in search of the sort of extreme cut their own hairdressers hesitated to provide.

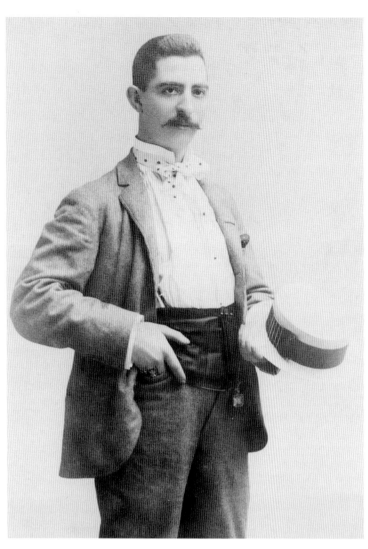

Pittsburgh, Pa., c.1900-1903

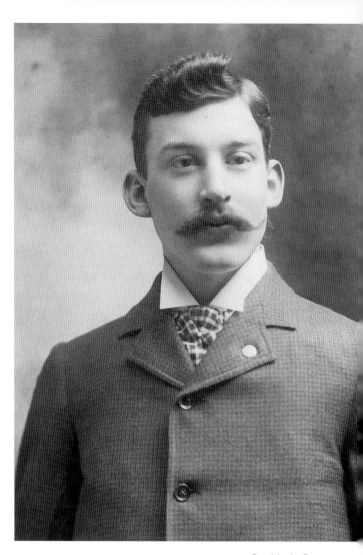

Braddock, Pa.,
c.1900-1902

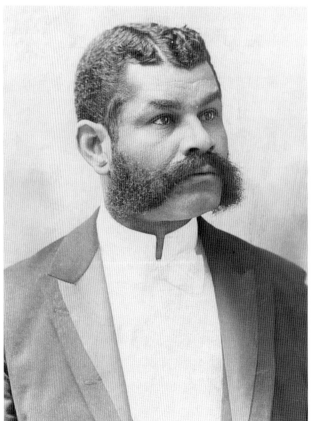

Philadelphia, Pa., dated 1902

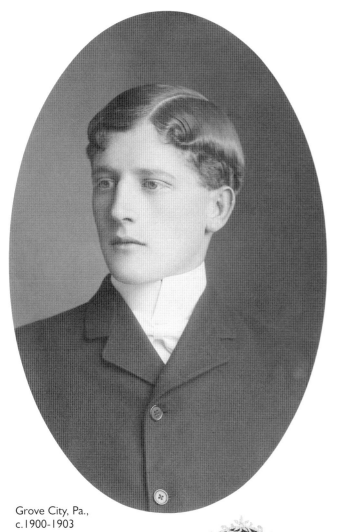

Grove City, Pa.,
c.1900-1903

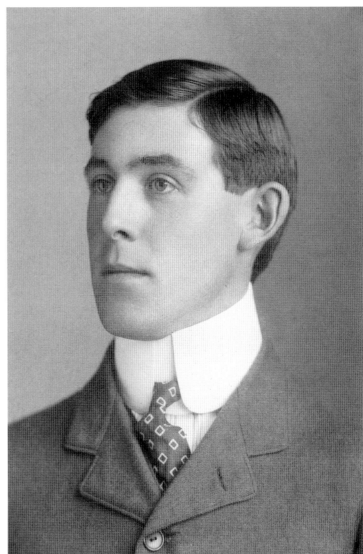

Meadville, Pa., c.1904-1906

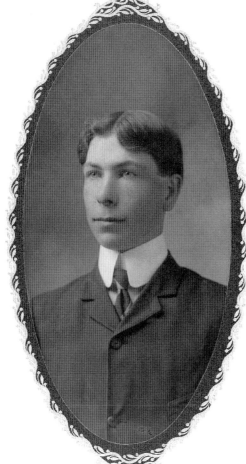

Punxsutawney, Pa., c.1905-1907

117

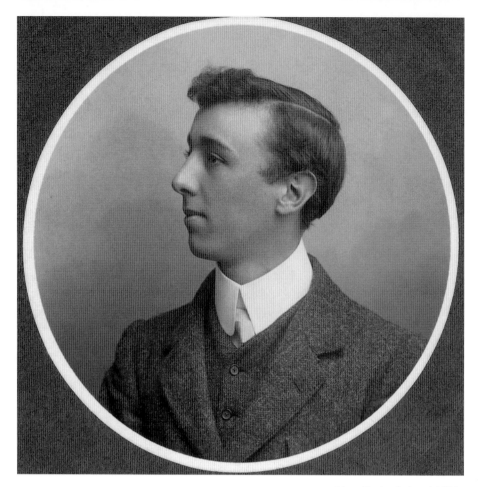

New England, dated 1906

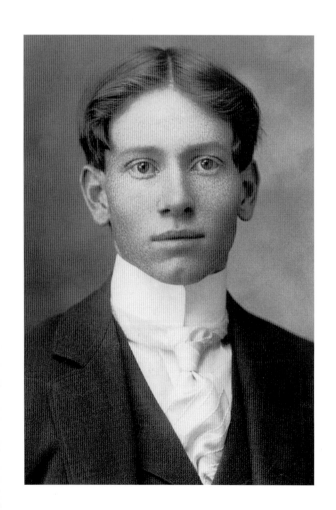

c.1906-1908

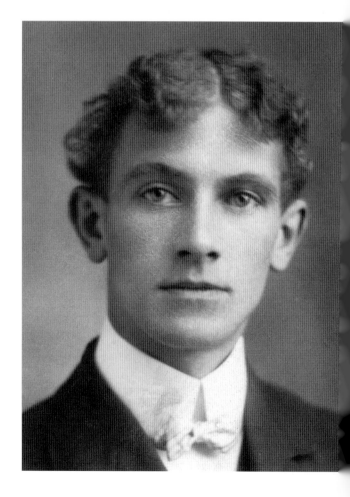

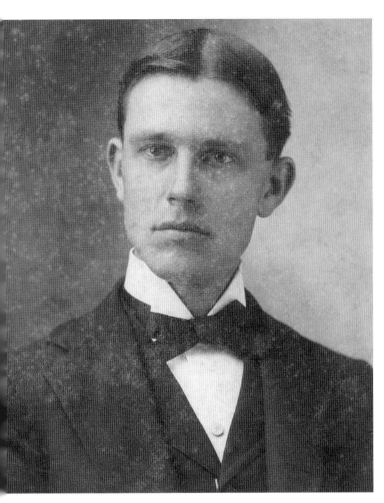
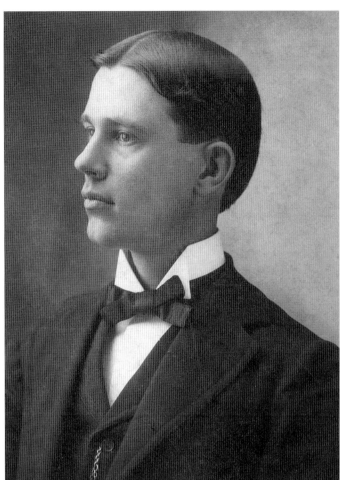

Tallassee, Ala., c.1906-1908

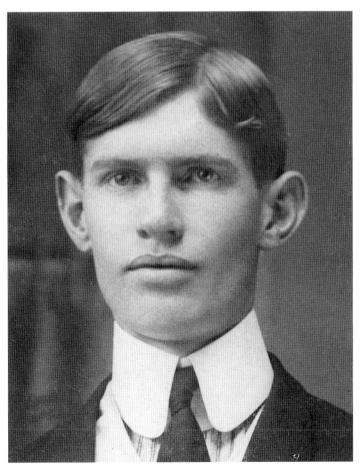

c.1910-1912

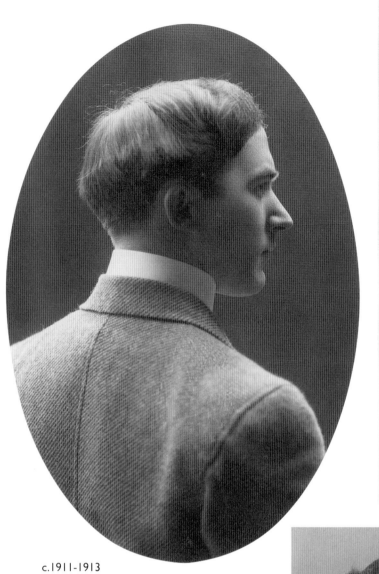

c.1911-1913

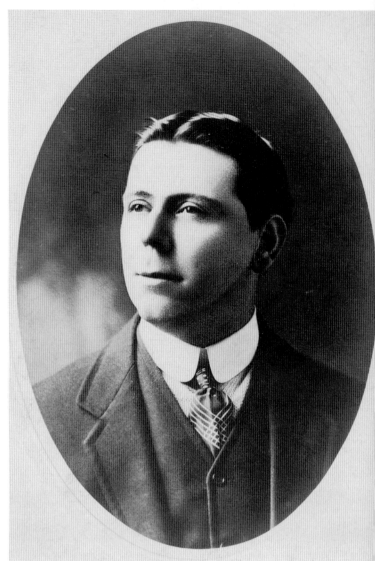

c.1910-1912

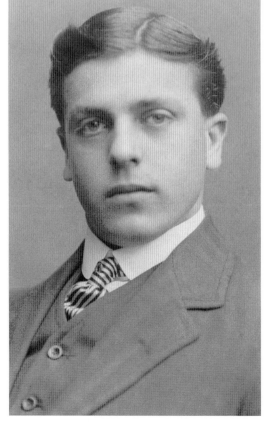

c.1910-1912

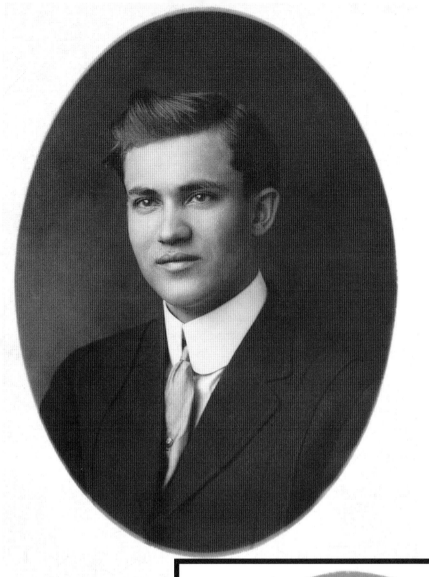

Mobile, Ala., dated 1914

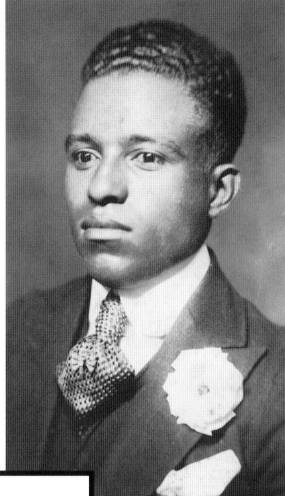

c.1910-1912

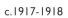

c.1917-1918

121

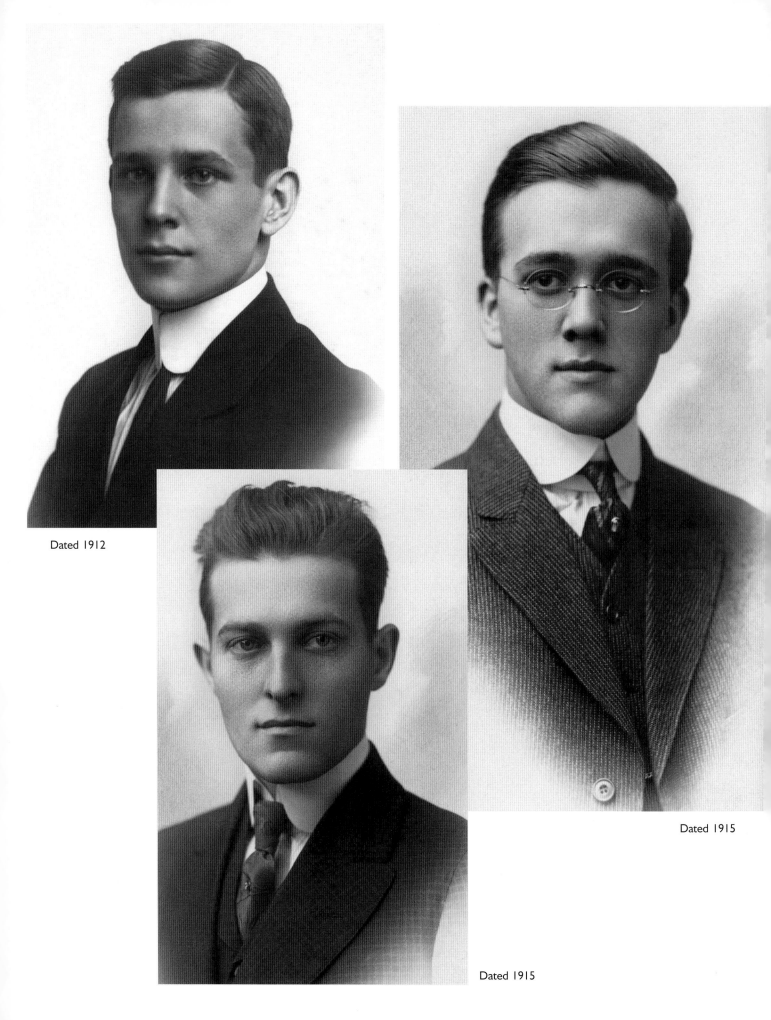

Dated 1912

Dated 1915

Dated 1915

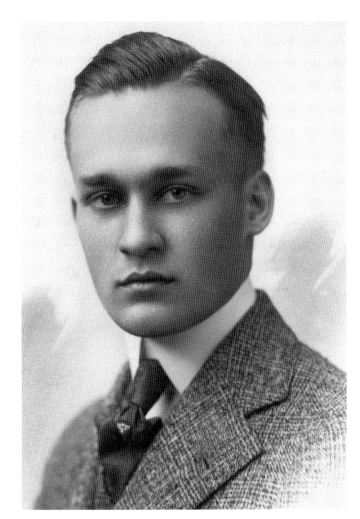

Dated 1915

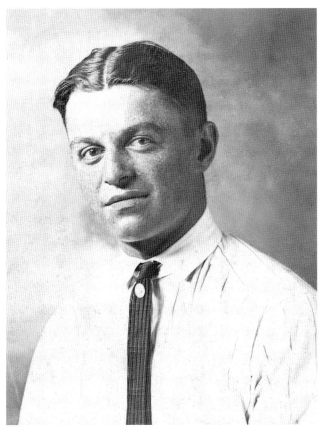

c.1918-1920

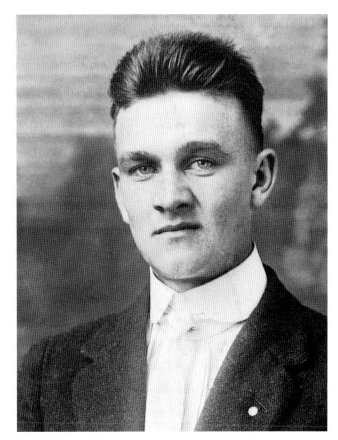

c.1920-1921

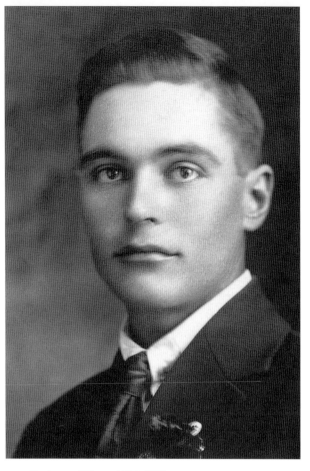

Markesan, Wis., c.1926-1928

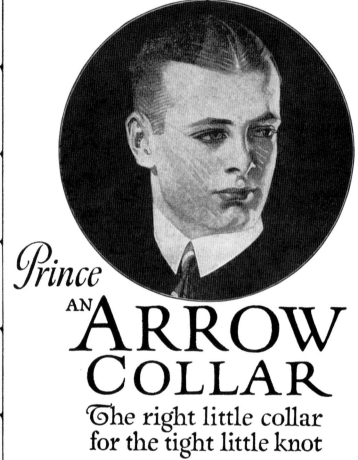

Prince
AN **ARROW COLLAR**
The right little collar
for the tight little knot

Cluett, Peabody & Co. Inc. MAKERS, *Troy, N.Y.*

FRD

The Arrow Collar man for 1920.

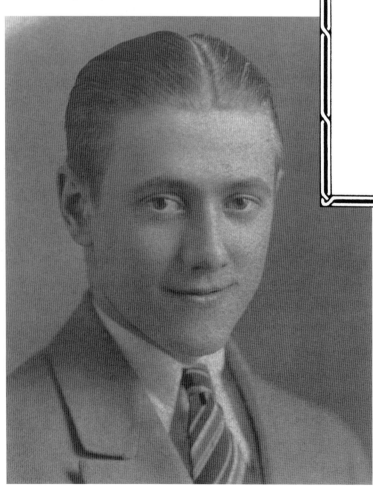

c.1925-1927

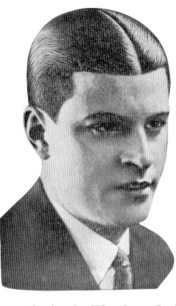

The Sport Cut

This cut is very popular with college men. It is parted in the middle and left full at the sides, using pomade to keep the hair back from the forehead.

Professional Trim

This trim is usually favored by men past forty years of age. The hair may be parted as desired. The beard should be tapered gradually into a graceful point by using clippers about three-quarters down the face and tapering the rest with shears.

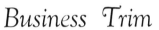

Business Trim

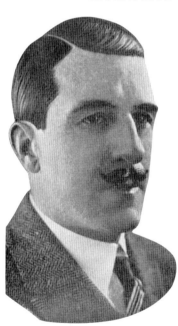

This trim is extremely well liked by the average business man. It is parted at the left side; cut into a featheredge effect at the neck, graduating gracefully toward the top. Avoid cutting too short.

Boyish Pompadour

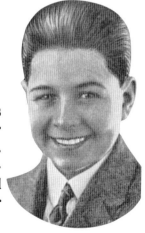

Practically all boys prefer to wear their hair in this style. It is cut in featheredge fashion, as in the sport cut, and combed straight back, using pomade to keep the hair in place.

Men and boys' styles for 1924 from *The Tonsorial Artist*.

Popular Hair Cut Styles for Men

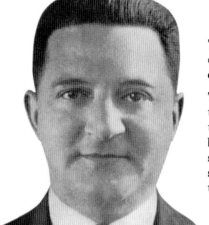

Short Pomp

This is a European style and the most difficult to cut. Pains should be taken to do it right.

The hair is cut into a featheredge finish at the neck and fairly short three-quarters up the back of the head. After cutting the back, brush the hair with a stiff brush and start cutting at the forehead to the desired length, working toward the back of the head, thus creating a hair brush effect.

Valentino

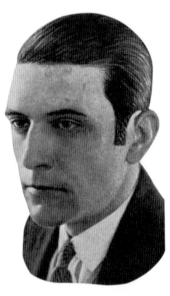

This cut is very becoming to young men of dark hair and complexion. The strong side beards are dropped heavy on the sides, ending slightly above the ear lobe. The hair is generally held back with pomade or other hair preparations. This cut may be parted on the side or brushed back. The back of the neck should be finished with a featheredge.

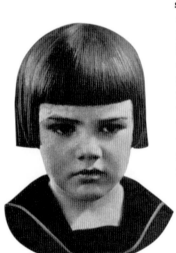

Buster Brown

This cut is very becoming to small boys between the age of four and seven years. It is cut as follows:

FIRST:—Part the hair in the middle and brush down firmly all around. Start the hair line at the tip of the ear lobe, exercising care to form a perfect, straight line all around the head. Taper the extreme edges with shears and comb as shown in Figure (2), page 22.

SECOND:—To form the bangs, brush the hair down on the forehead, starting about one inch above the hair line. Cut a perfect straight line from temple to temple about three-eighths of an inch above the eyebrows, creating the effect shown in the above photograph.

Men and boys' styles for 1924 from *The Tonsorial Artist*.

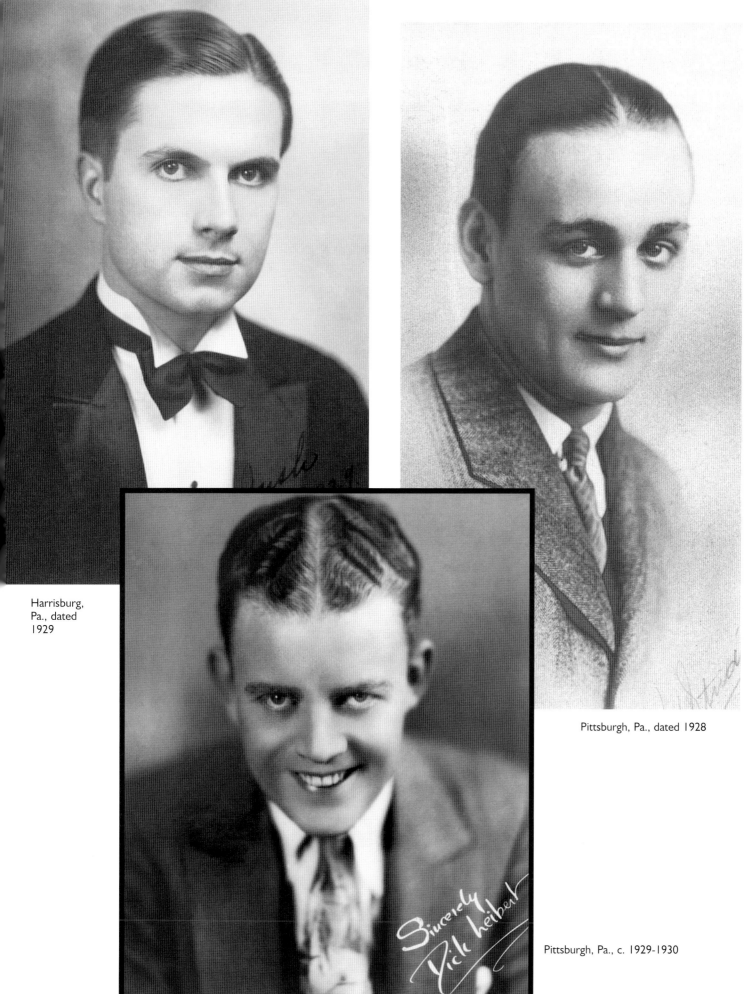

Harrisburg,
Pa., dated
1929

Pittsburgh, Pa., dated 1928

Pittsburgh, Pa., c. 1929-1930

127

Chapter Four
In Mama's and Papa's Image

Children's Hair: Introduction

"For little girls there is nothing particularly new, they are their mammas in miniature," *Godey's Lady's Book* declared in 1867. The same could have been said about the preceding decades, and it could just as easily have been applied to boys as well as girls. Little boys of the 1830s and 1840s were almost indistinguishable from their sisters in clothing and hairstyle. It was well into the 20th century before boys were completely free of skirts and long curls. Curls, in fact, were a source of childhood misery for both sexes.

Bouncing ringlets on childish heads were always a delight—and where nature fell short a determined mother often stepped in. Elisabeth McClellan noted that "curl papers were the torment of almost every little girl in the nursery." Even false hair was added during periods when fashion demanded excess. Some doting mothers of the 1870s took matters to further extremes, holding "hops," which were society balls in exact replica.

The editor of *Harper's Monthly* joined an audience of preening parents to witness one of these events in 1873. He was horrified to see the gowned, waistcoated and coifed children copy not only the dances of their parents, but their gossipy pettiness and snobbery as well. "It was certainly pretty, but it was a very sober spectacle," he wrote, finding the whole affair unforgivable.

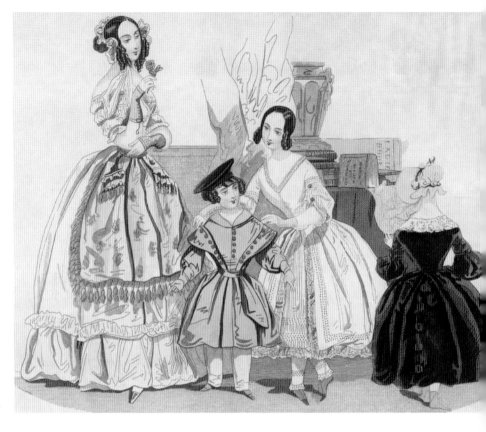

Godey's Lady's Book, 1841
A child's hair was an imitation of the adult. Even boys wore curls like mama.

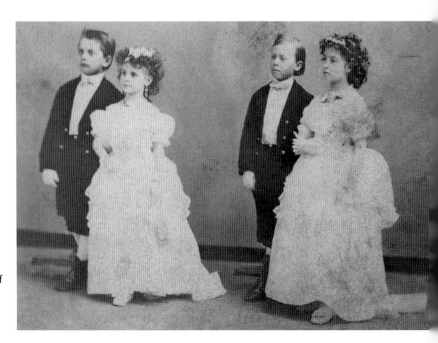

Mansfield, Ohio, c.1873
Rare photograph of participants in a children's hop.

Fortunately the average mother was content to allow her children to be children. Girls' locks were given their freedom until the age of eight or nine, after which a subdued version of fashionable restraints was applied. For boys it was much the same. Baby curls were clipped before a son went off to school for the first time, and the rule of "like father like son" prevailed.

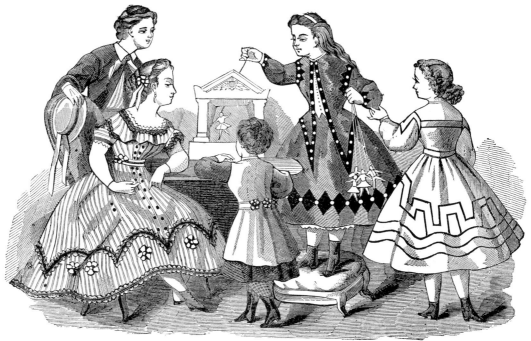

CHILDREN'S FASHIONS FOR MAY

The fashion for children in 1867 from *Peterson's Magazine*.

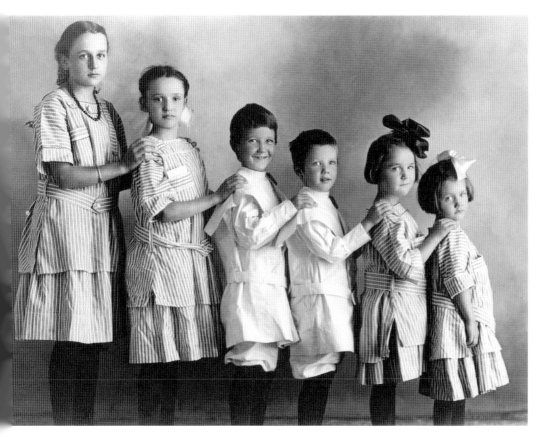

The fashion for children c.1916-1918.

Girls

Girls were especially subject to the whims and fads of the adult world. The sausage-like curls that hung in unnatural bunches from women's heads from the 1840s into the 1860s were reproduced on their daughters. After the age of eight or nine a girl could expect to have her hair pulled back as severely as her mother's for daytime, or restrained in a snood-like net.

Decorative combs and ornaments held together uncomfortable chignons and twists for the child of fashion during the 1870s and 1880s. Ribbons and bows were, by comparison, a welcome and attractive styling aid until their sheer size made them a torment in the 20th century. Girls' parts remained in the center until the late 1870s.

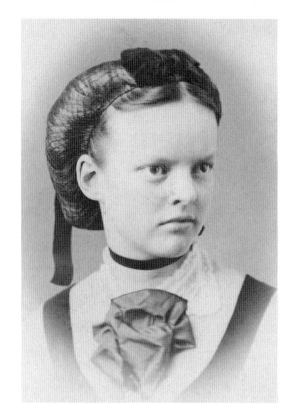

Nets were an unnatural and uncomfortable hair accessory for girls well into the early 1870s.

Certain hair fashions remained constant for girls, regardless of other trends. Braids were worn singly and in pairs, wrapped around the head and in coils. Bangs that were shaped ear to ear in the 1880s were being cut straight across by the 1890s or were absorbed into frizz, only to reappear straight and smooth in the early 1900s.

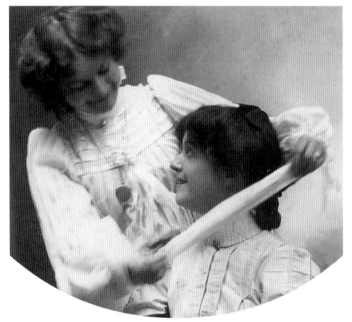

Adding the hair ribbon, c.1905.

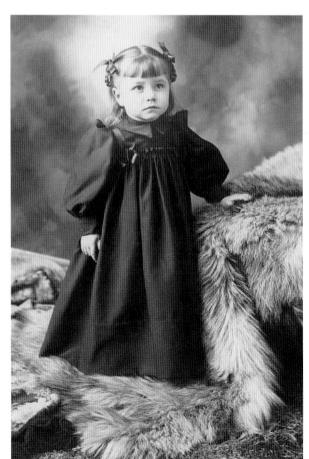

Bangs cut straight across, a loop of braids on each side, and bows for decoration in 1897.

The modern bob was a blessing for little girls who were allowed to wear it. But too many mothers still meddled, as they always had, curl papers and heated tongs in hand. They had yet to learn the valuable lesson that the best and most attractive fashion choice a mother could make for a daughter was to let her hair fall loose and natural.

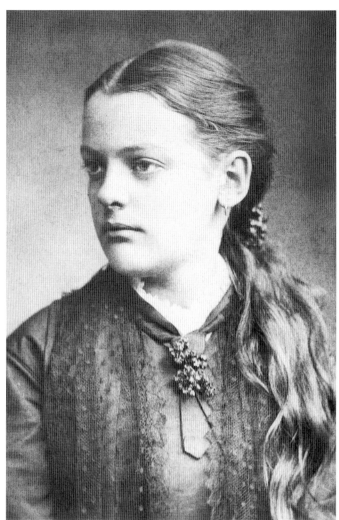

c.1880-1882
A natural fall of hair was always the best complement to youthful beauty.

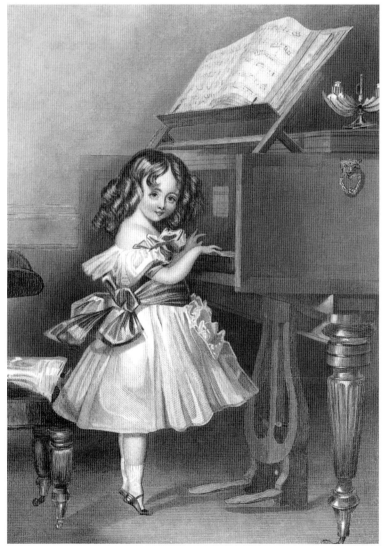

The Lady's Companion, 1842

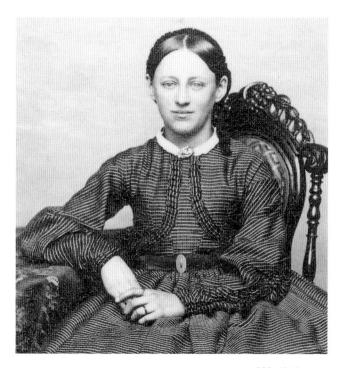

c.1859-1860

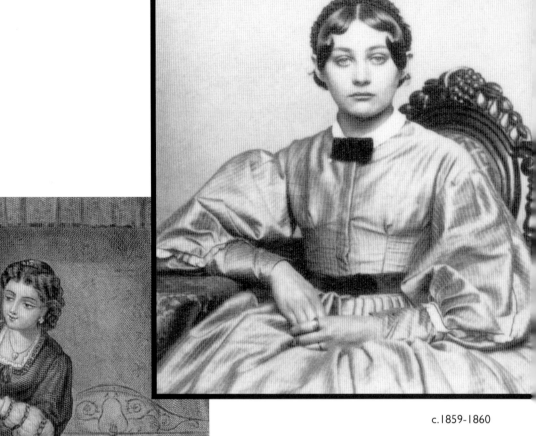

c.1859-1860

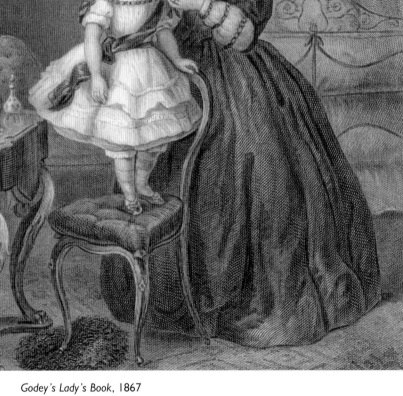

Godey's Lady's Book, 1867

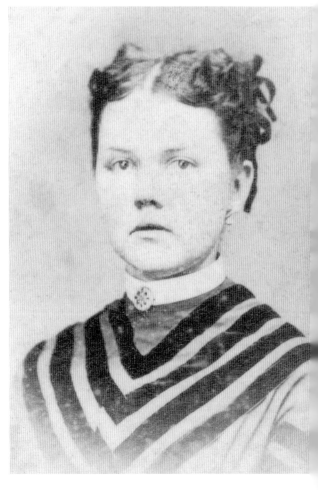

St. Louis, Mo., dated 1862

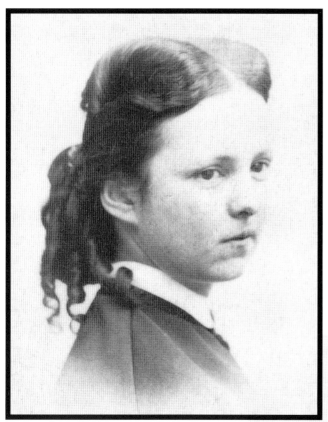

Lowell, Mass., c.1864-1866

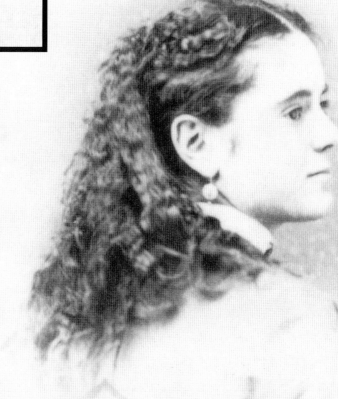

Baldwinsville, N.Y., c.1866-1868

Farmer Village, N.Y., c. 1867-1869

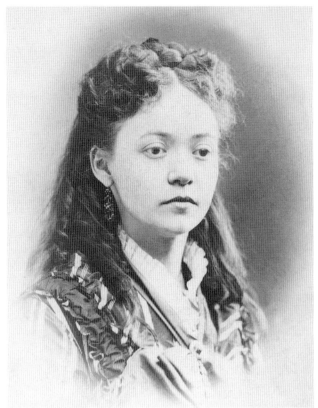

Sterling, Ill., c.1877-1879

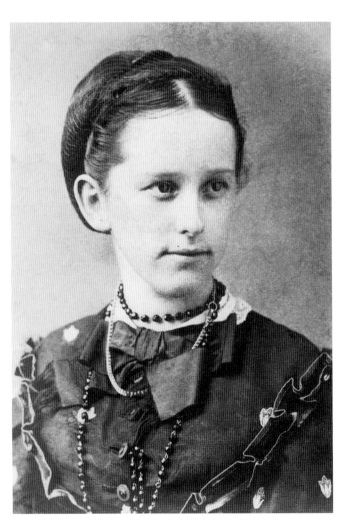

Bridgewater, Mass., c.1872-1874

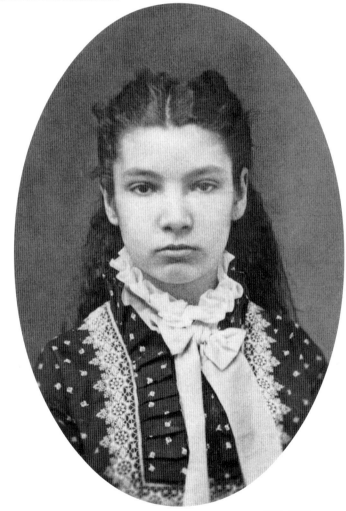

c.1875-1876

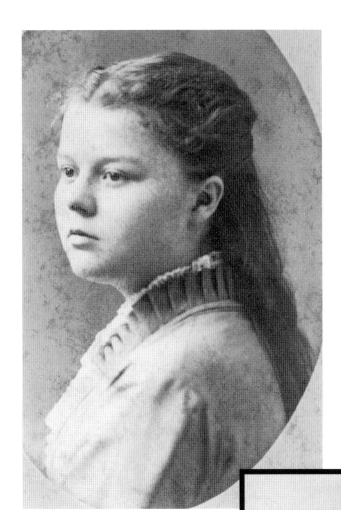

Sinclearville, Ill., c. 1877-1879

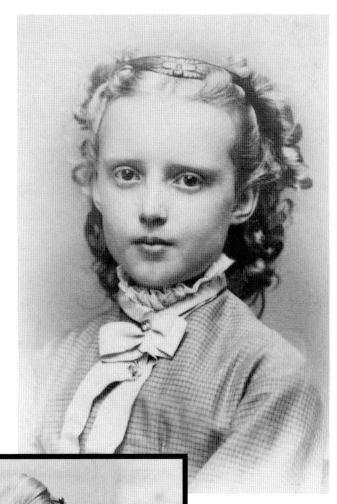

Rochester, Minn., c.1878-1880

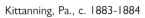

Kittanning, Pa., c. 1883-1884

135

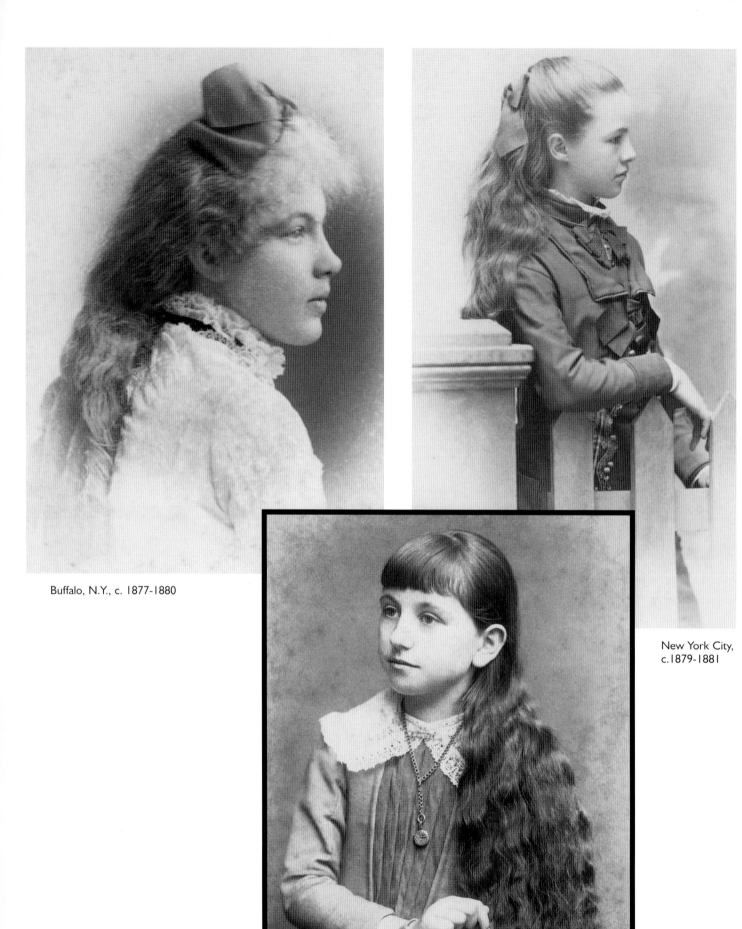

Buffalo, N.Y., c. 1877-1880

New York City,
c.1879-1881

Lebanon, Pa., c. 1883-1885

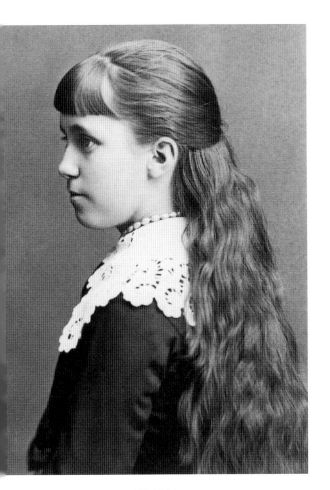

Waltham, Mass., c.1882-1884

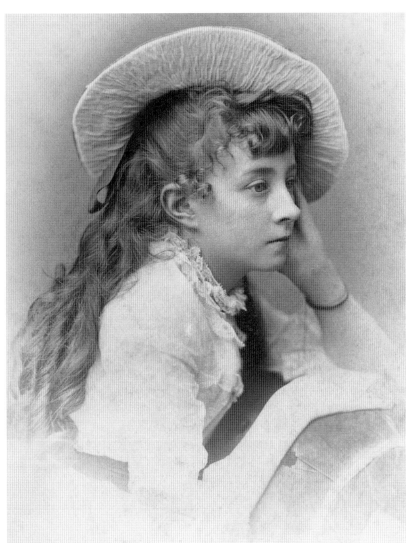

Bridgeport, Conn., c.1884-1888

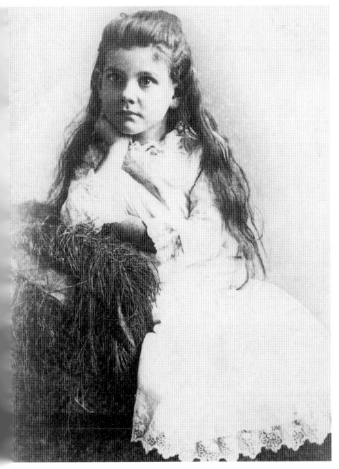

Decatur, Ill., c.1883-1885

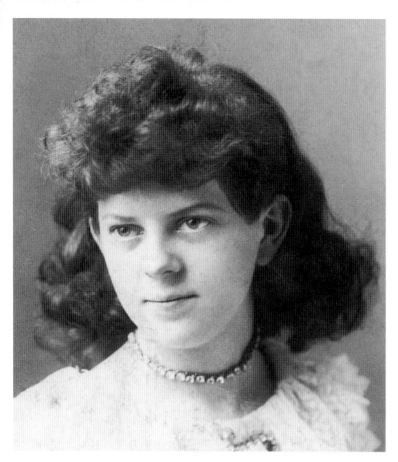

New York City, c.1890-1892

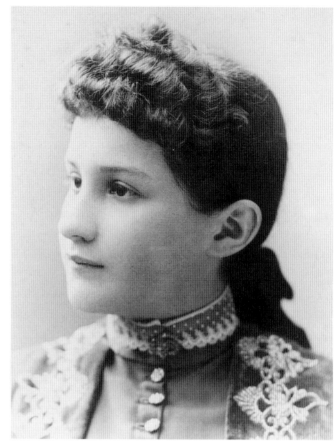

York, Pa., c. 1887-1889

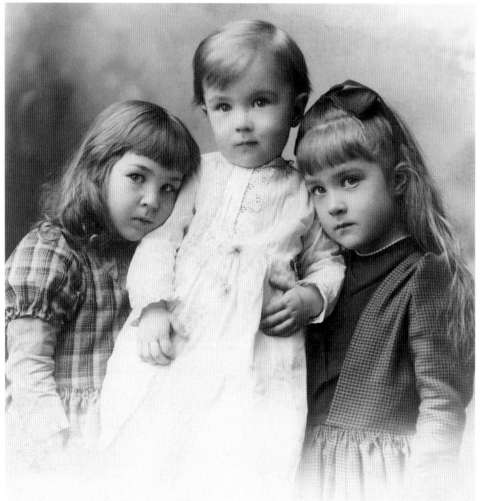

Lowell, Mass., c.1892-1894

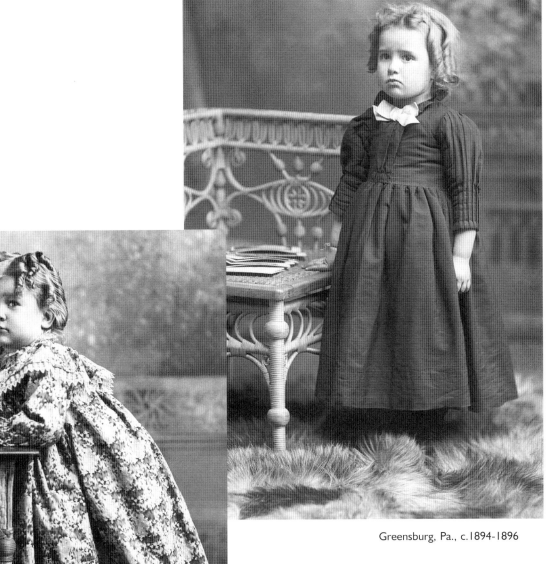

Greensburg, Pa., c.1894-1896

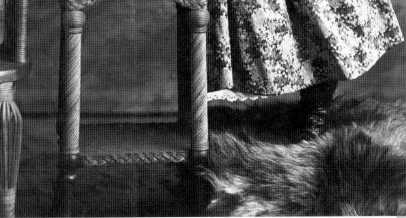

Cumberland, Md., dated 1896

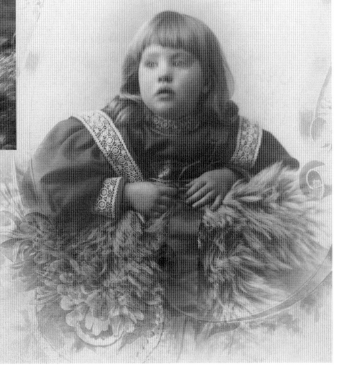

Keyser, W.Va., c.1894-1896

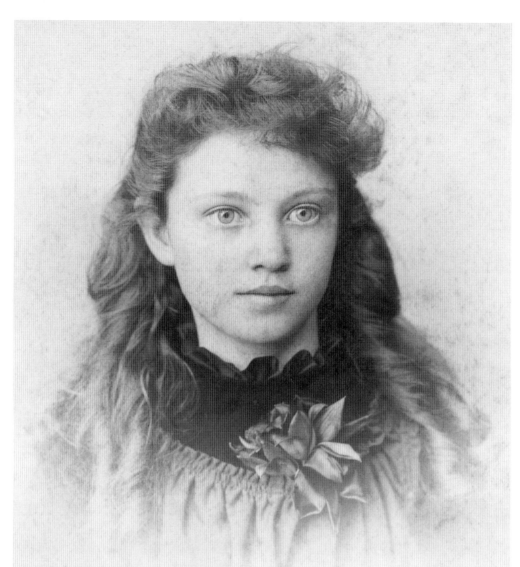

Emlenton, Pa.,
c.1898-1900

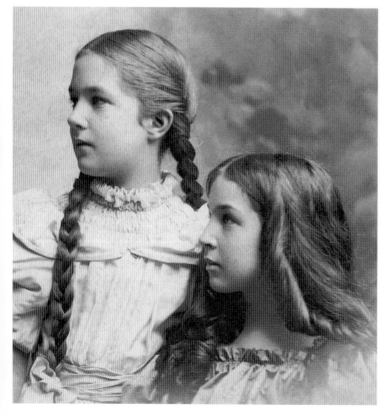

Lowell, Mass., c.1900

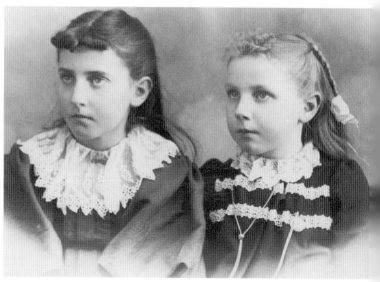

Weyauwega, Wis., c.1898-1900

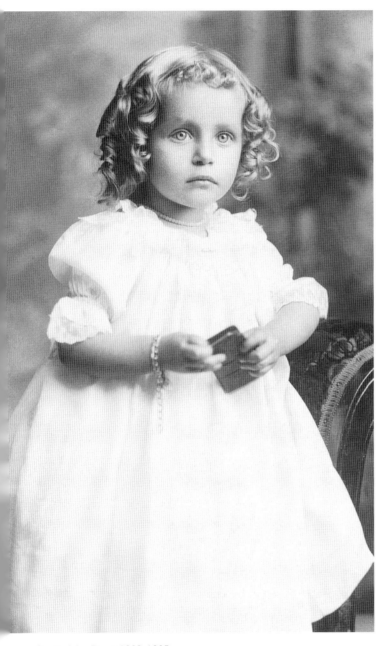

Scottsdale, Pa., c.1903-1905

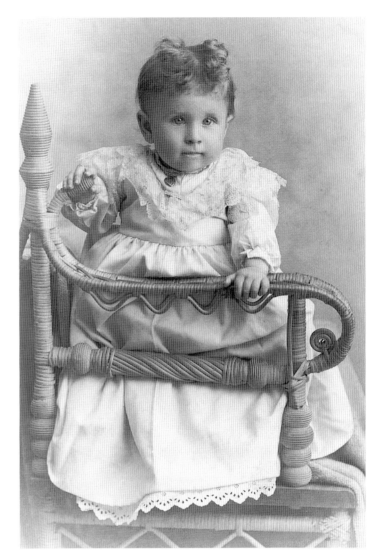

Bellevue, Ohio, c.1900-1903

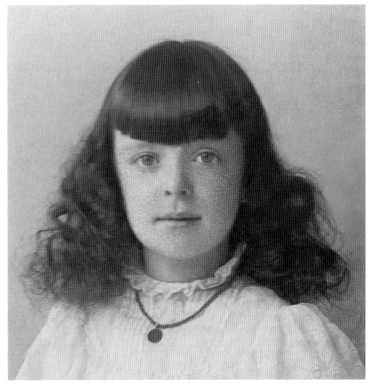

Bridgeport, Conn., c.1903-1905

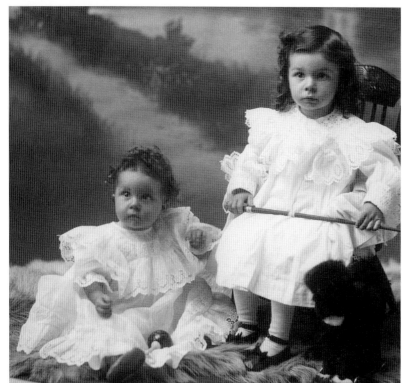

Kane. Pa., c.1905-1908

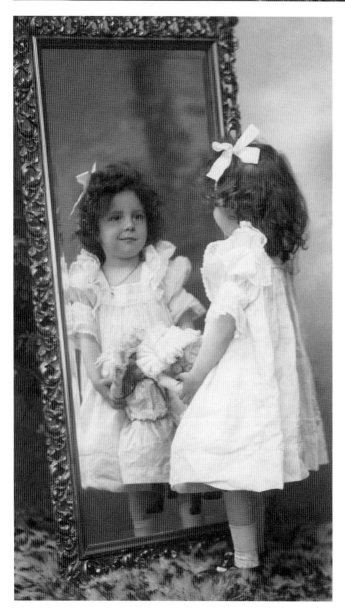

Kane, Pa., c.1908-1910

c.1904-1906

142

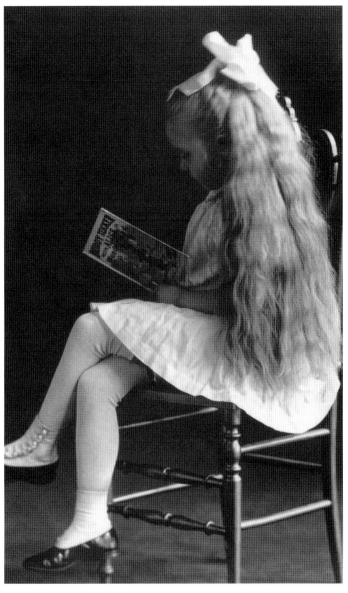

c.1910-1912

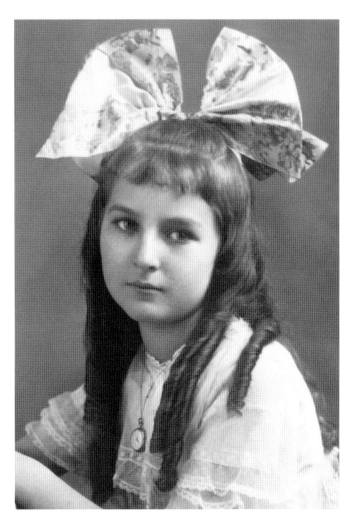

c.1910-1912

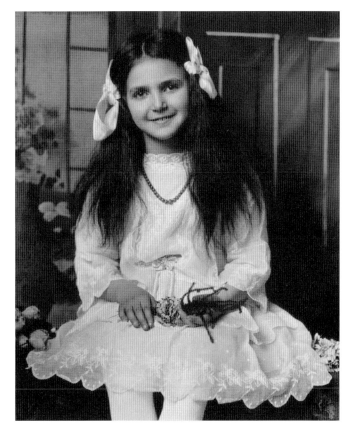

c.1909-1911

143

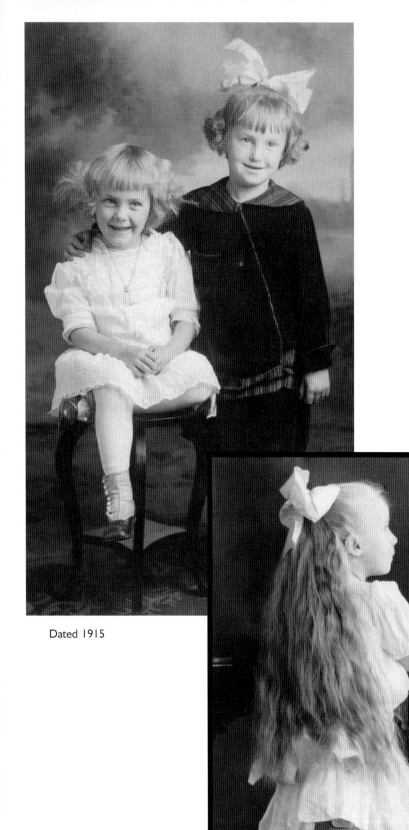

Dated 1915

c.1910-1912

ARRANGING YOUR LITTLE GIRL'S HAIR
By Ida C. Van Auken

At Three a Narrow Ribbon is Worn

Wider Ribbon is Used for an Older Child

Direct Center Parting With All-Around Band

The Ladies' Home Journal, 1916

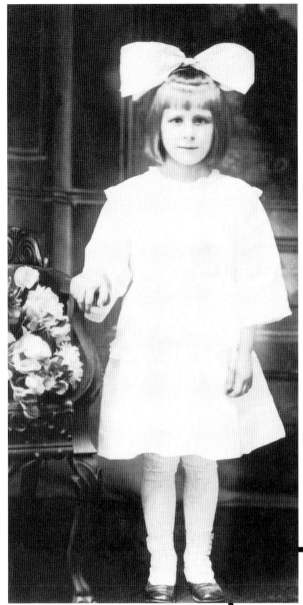

Waterbury, Conn., c.1919-1920

Leechburg, Pa., c. 1923-1925

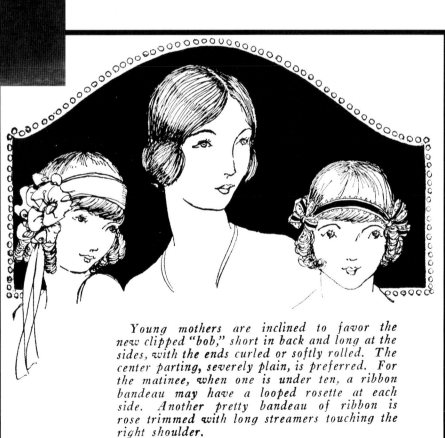

Young mothers are inclined to favor the new clipped "bob," short in back and long at the sides, with the ends curled or softly rolled. The center parting, severely plain, is preferred. For the matinee, when one is under ten, a ribbon bandeau may have a looped rosette at each side. Another pretty bandeau of ribbon is rose trimmed with long streamers touching the right shoulder.

Today's Housewife, 1923

Daddy

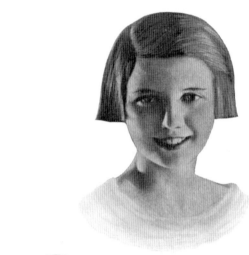

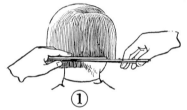
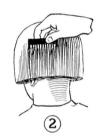

This style is prevalent among very young school girls, between the ages of 10 and 14 years. It should be cut as follows:

First:—Part the hair at the side and brush down firmly all around. Start the hair line parallel with the ear lobe, and cut perfectly straight all around by holding the shears and comb as shown in figure (1). After the hair is bobbed, it should be brushed back from the forehead slightly and worn with a barrette or comb, as shown in figure (2).

Remove fuzzy hair from the neck up to the hair line, with fine sharp clippers.

When the bob is finished, it should look exactly like the central figure.

The time required to complete this bob, should not exceed fifteen (15) minutes.

Above and right:
The Tonsorial Artist, 1924

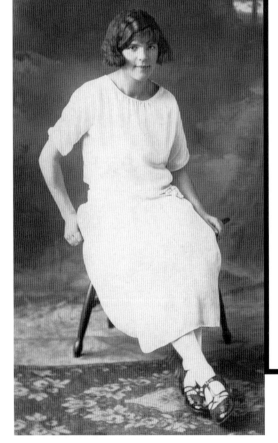

c.1924-1926

Diella

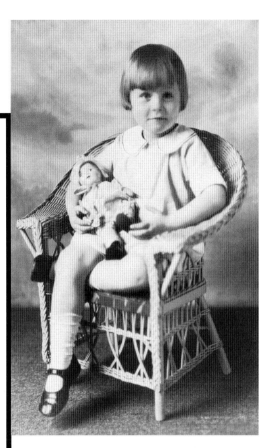

c.1928-1930

This style is very pretty on small girls, who have straight hair and wear it curled at the sides. It should be cut as follows:

FIRST:—Part the hair in the middle and brush it down smoothly. Start the hair line parallel with the ear lobe, and shingle back just as you would in a Boyish Bob, with graduating shortness as shown in figure (1).

SECOND:—To form the bangs, brush the hair down on the forehead about one inch from the hair line. Cut straight from temple to temple directly above the eyebrows. Brush the hair carefully several times, wetting it if necessary. See that the bangs are perfectly straight by holding your shears in position as shown in figure (2).

When the bob is finished, it should be curled at the sides to obtain the desired effect, as shown in the central figure.

The time required to complete this bob, including the curling, should not exceed thirty-five (35) minutes.

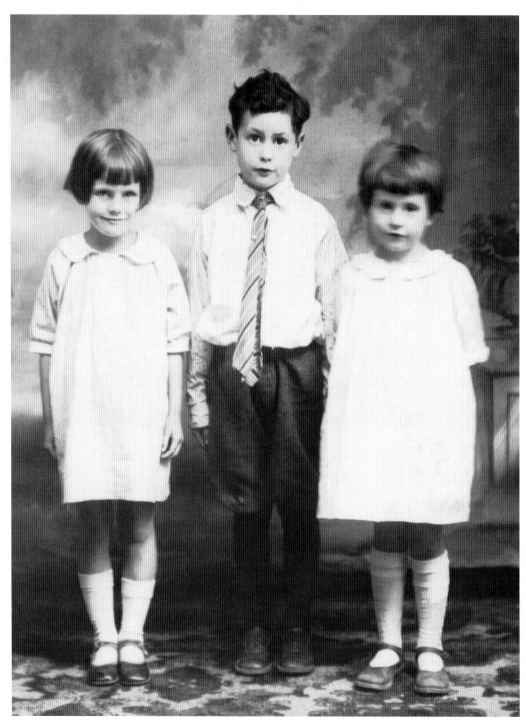

c.1928-1930

Boys

Most boys wore varying amounts of hair until the age of six or seven, when father took charge and the barber was consulted. From that point on they were truly their papa's image, adopting the accepted style for the time. Parts were a particular matter of concern. Boys' parts remained on the side until men began dividing their hair in the center in the mid-1870s. Even then the center part was resisted by boys who considered it girlish, and by parents who feared their infant sons would be mistaken for daughters

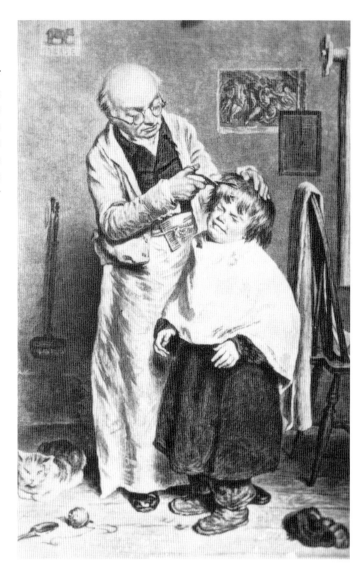

The first haircut was a rite of passage from infancy to boyhood.

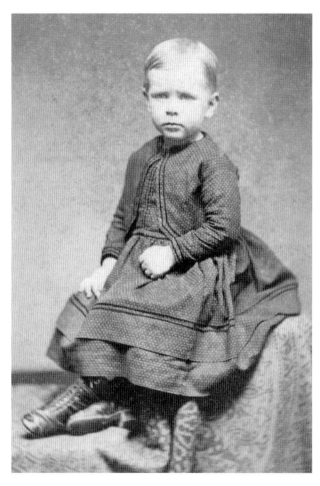

His side part gives away the fact that this c.1864 toddler is a boy.

The practice of draping small boys in ringlets had nearly died out when Frances Hodgson Burnett published her novel, *Little Lord Fauntleroy*, in 1886. She described her young hero as a "graceful, childish figure in a black velvet suit, with a lace collar, and with lovelocks waving about the handsome, manly little face." The effect on American mothers was electric.

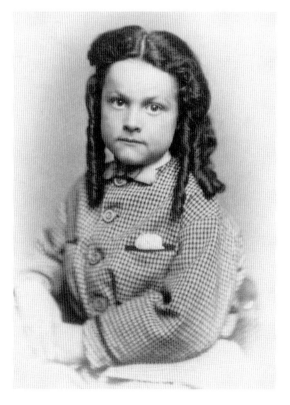

Long curls weren't uncommon in the late 1860s.

Women's magazines published patterns for the outfit, dry goods stores could barely keep in a supply of velveteen, and little boys were forbidden the barbershop. The trend was further energized when touring companies took a stage version of the book to every place large enough to own an opera house or town hall.

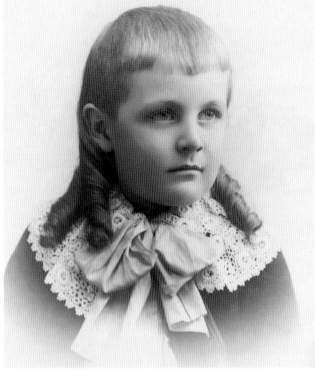

The curse of Little Lord Fauntleroy even reached Grand Forks, N.D. in the late 1880s.

"Beaver Dam's citizens waded knee-deep in Fauntleroys—tall and short, lean and fat, freckled, snub-nosed and bespectacled," Harlowe Randall Hoyt remembered in his 1955 book *Town Hall Tonight*. He described with disgust his own mother's attempts to twist his hair into dangling ringlets. Hoyt ended the ordeal with a pair of stolen sewing scissors, but others continued to suffer the curse of Little Lord Fauntleroy well into the 1920s.

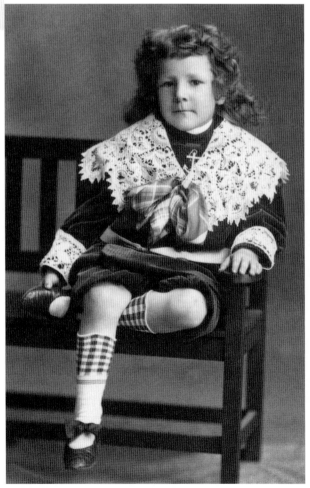

Curls too precious to be cut still plagued boys of the early 1900s.

150

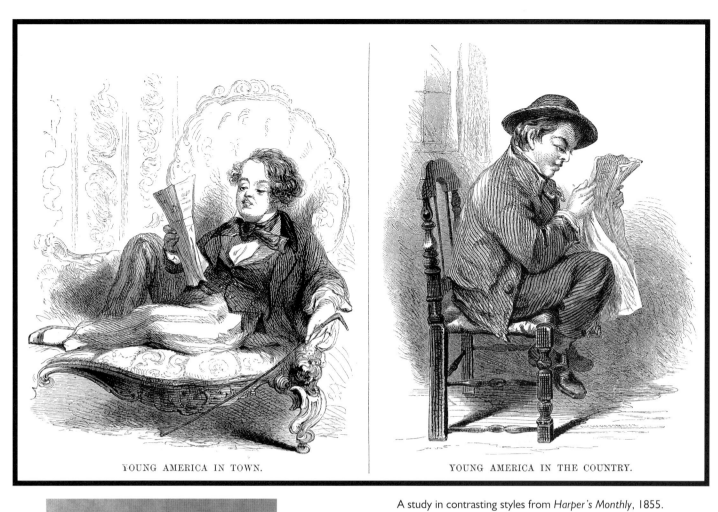

YOUNG AMERICA IN TOWN.

YOUNG AMERICA IN THE COUNTRY.

A study in contrasting styles from *Harper's Monthly*, 1855.

DeKalb, Ill., c. 1860-1862

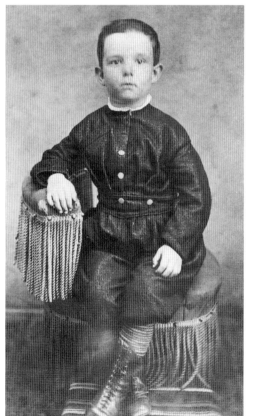

c.1862-1864

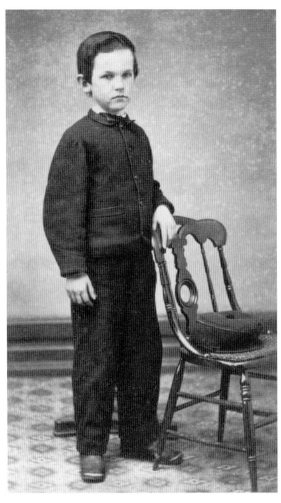

Farmer, N.Y., c.1863-1865

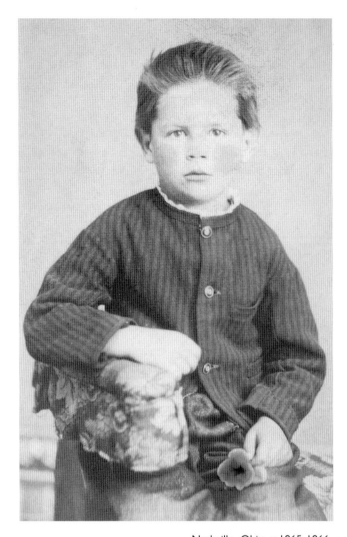

Nashville, Ohio, c.1865-1866

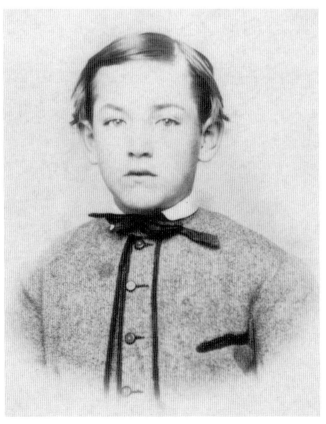

Baldwinsville, N.Y.,
c.1863-1865

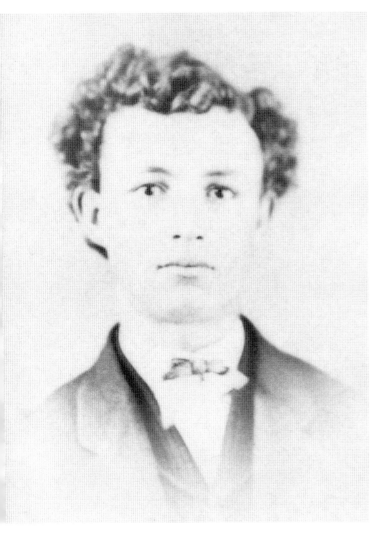

Newton, Pa., c. 1865-1868

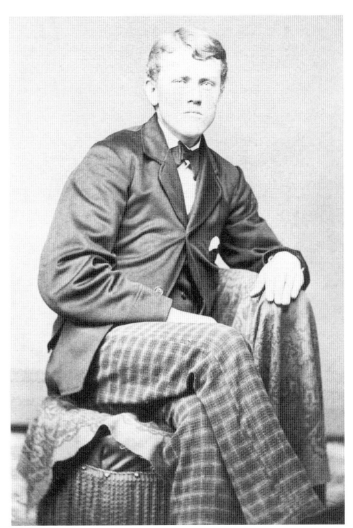

Bloomfield, Pa., c. 1869-1870

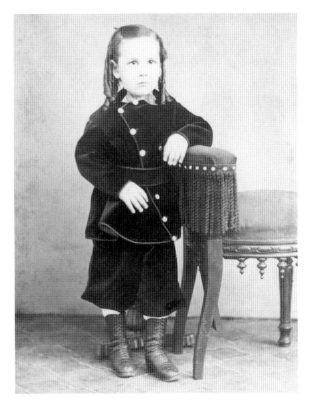

Boston, Mass., c.1869-1870

153

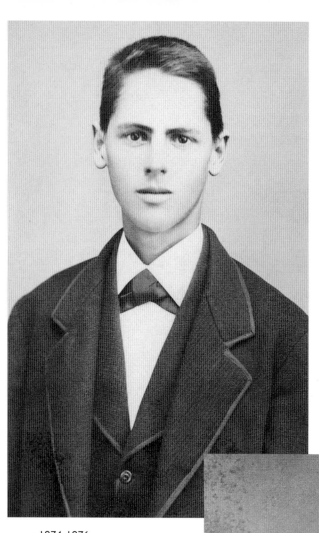

c.1874-1876

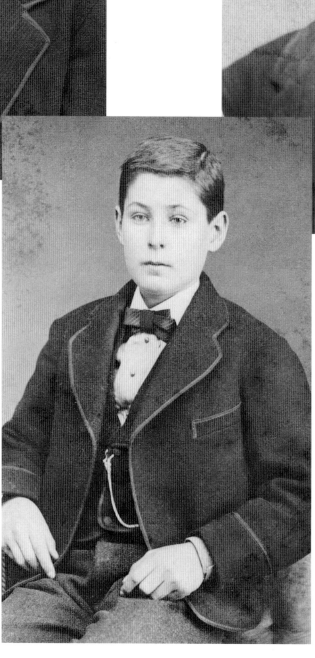

Newark, Ohio, c.1873-1874

Des Moines, Iowa,
c.1875-1877

154

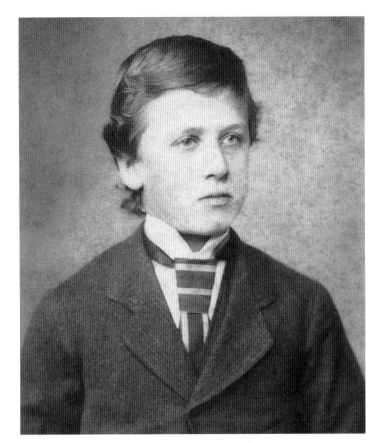

Lancaster, Pa., c.1878-1881

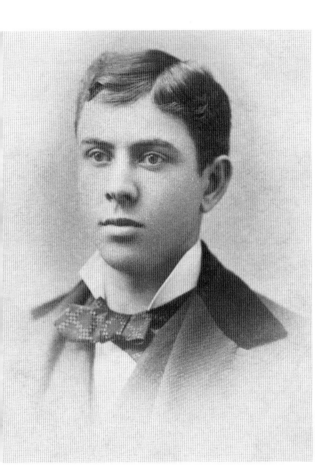

Titusville, Pa., c.1877-1880

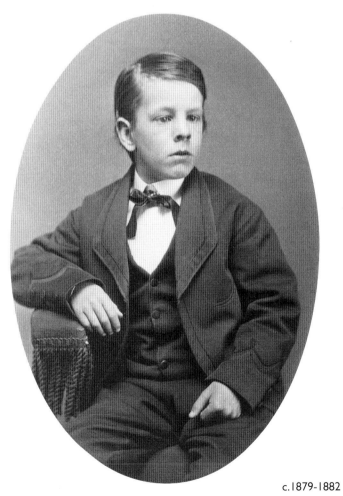

c.1879-1882

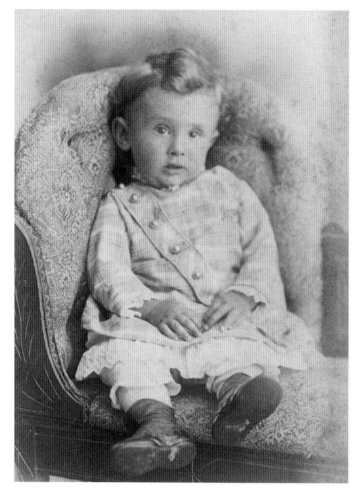

Emporia, Kans., c.1881-1883

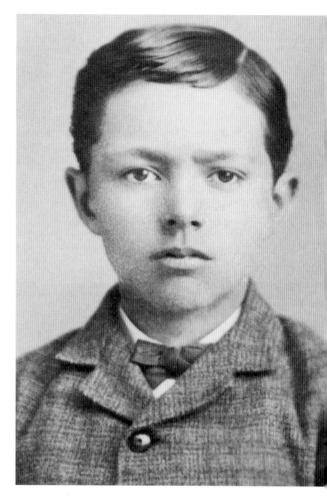

Greenfield, Mass., c. 1880-1883

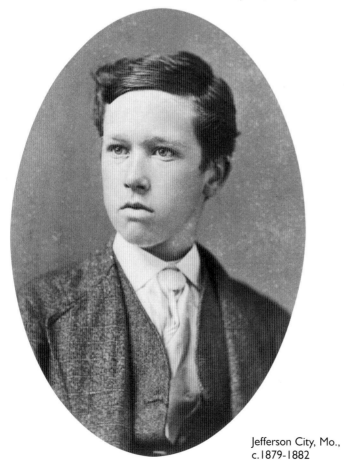

Jefferson City, Mo.,
c.1879-1882

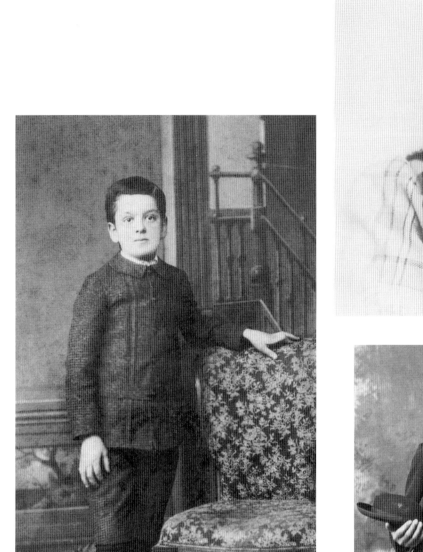

York, Pa., c.1886-1888

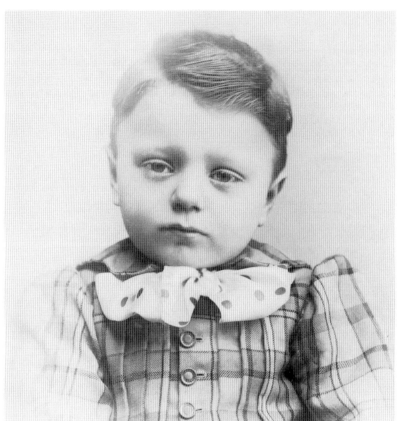

Winchester, Ind.,
c.1888-1890

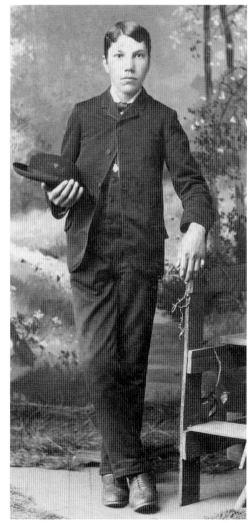

Pittsburgh, Pa.,
c.1888-1890

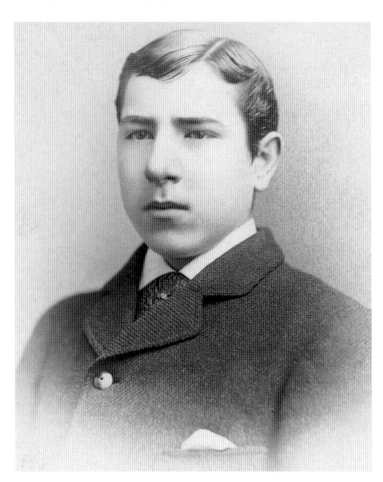

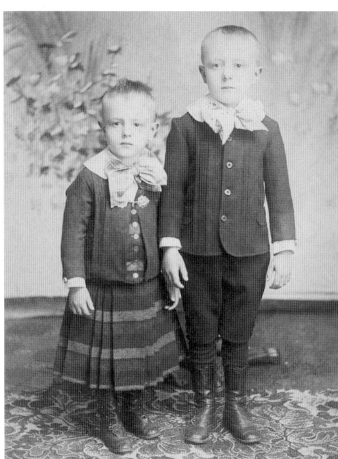

Albany, N.Y., c.1890-1892

Butler, Pa., c. 1890-1892

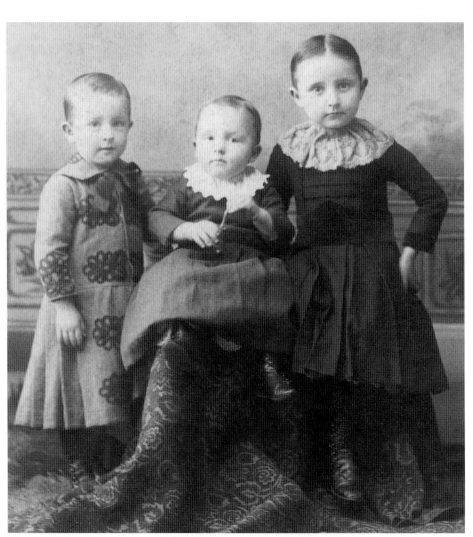

Owasso, Mich., c.1892-1894

158

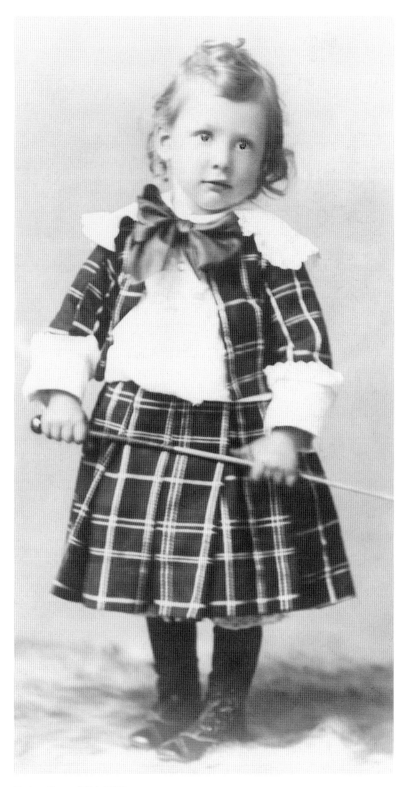

Butler, Pa., c.1894-1896

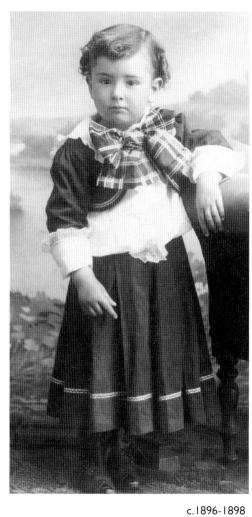

c.1896-1898

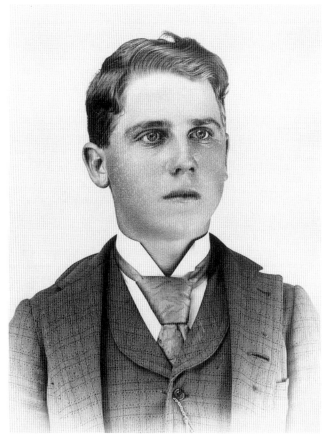

Dayton, Pa., c.1894-1896

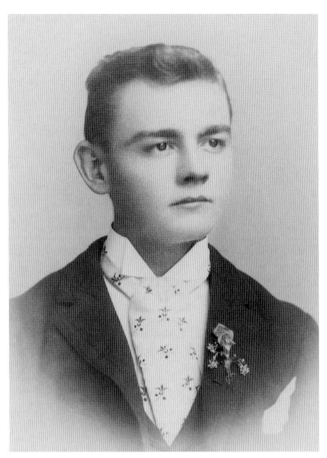

Hanover, Pa., c.1898-1899

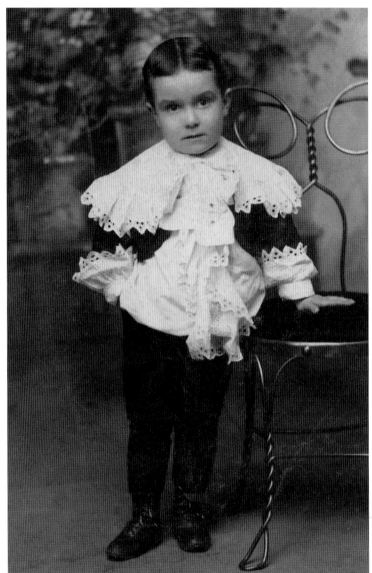

Jackson, Mich., c.1898-1901

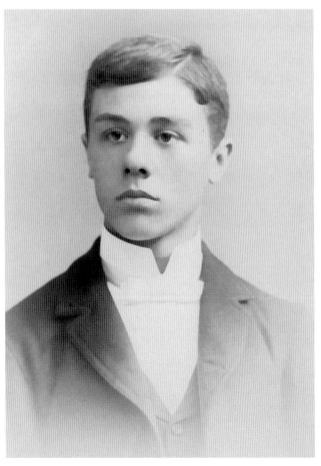

York, Pa., c.1897-1900

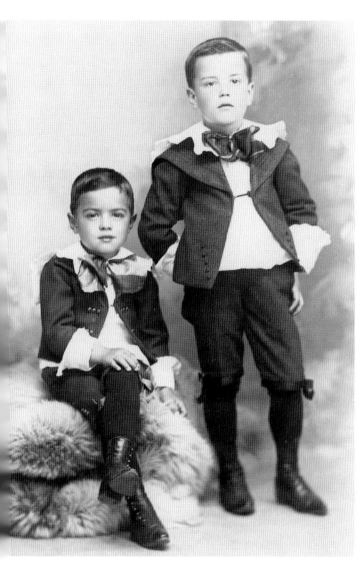

New Kensington, Pa., 1897-1900

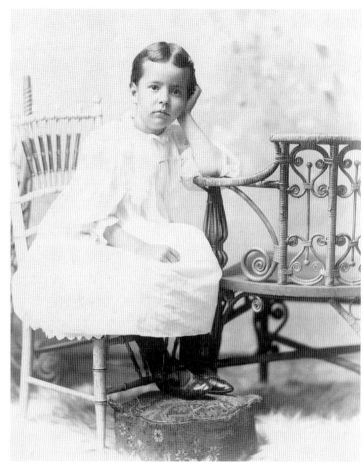

Springfield, Mass., dated 1897

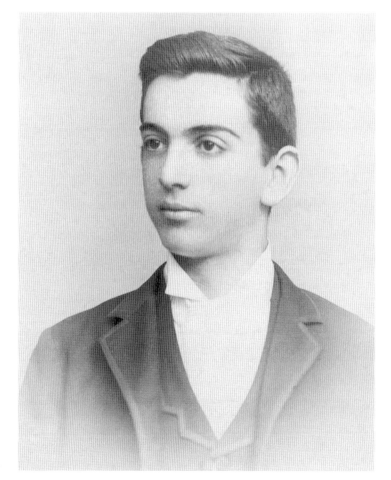

York, Pa., c.1900-1902

161

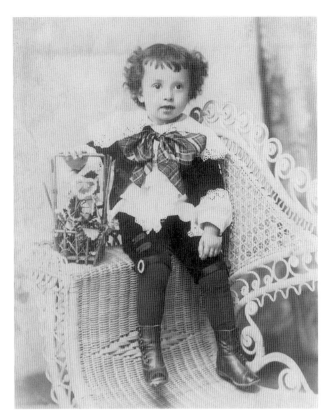

Philadelphia, Pa., c.1900-1903

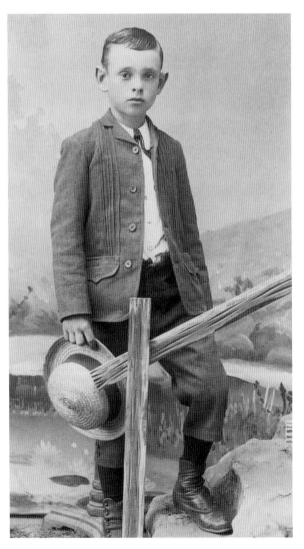

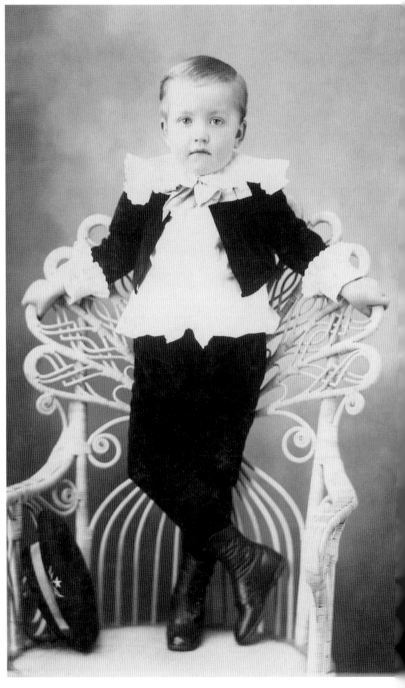

c.1900-1903

Staunton, Va., c.1903-1906

162

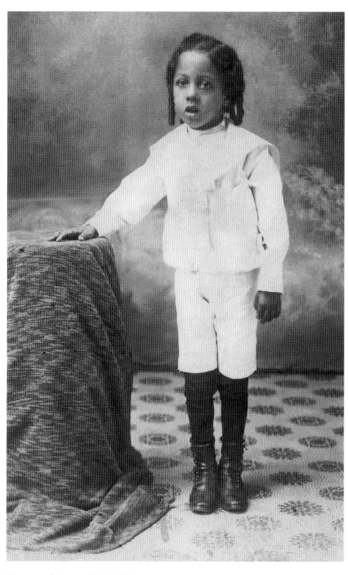

Dayton, Ohio, c.1905-1907

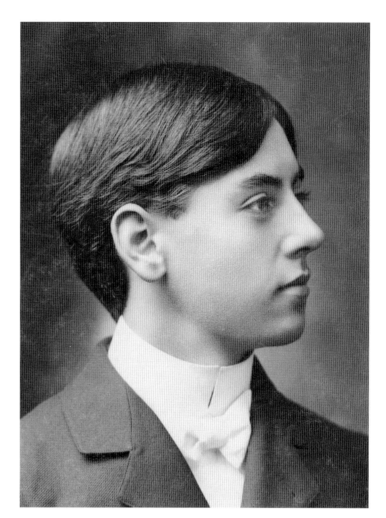

Mt. Pleasant, Pa., c.1905-1906

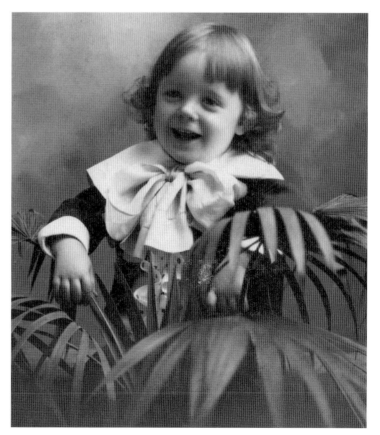

St. Louis, Mo., c.1905-1906

163

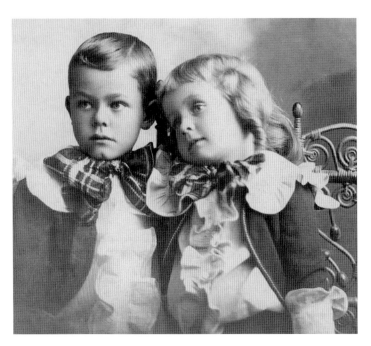

c. 1904-1906

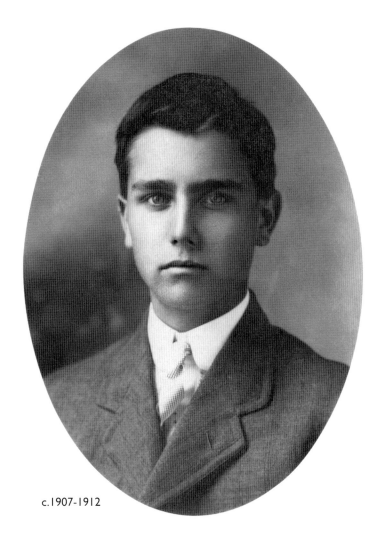

c. 1907-1912

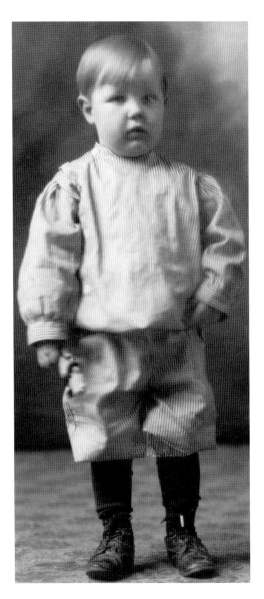

Salina, Pa.,
dated
1908

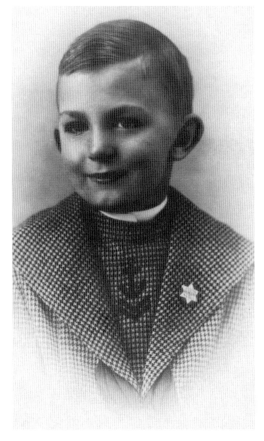

Cleveland,
Ohio,
dated 1908

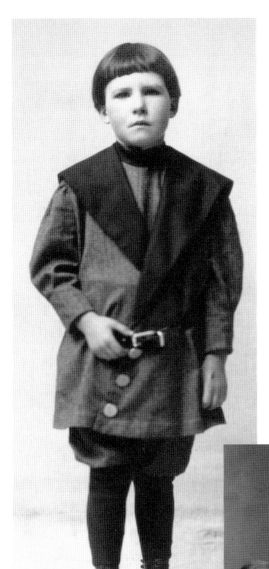

c.1909-1912

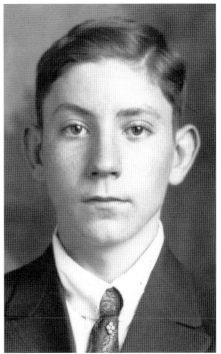

c.1913-1916

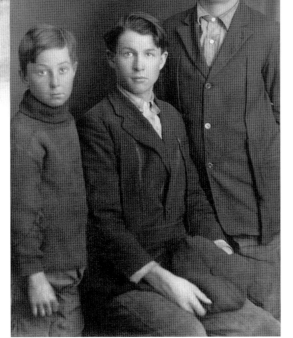

c.1915-1918

c.1915-1917

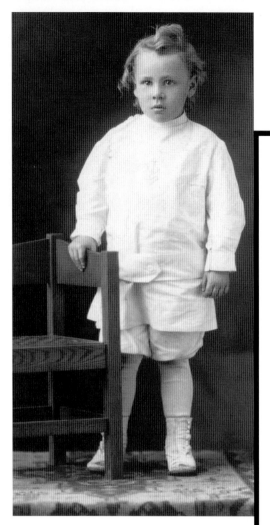

c.1912-1916

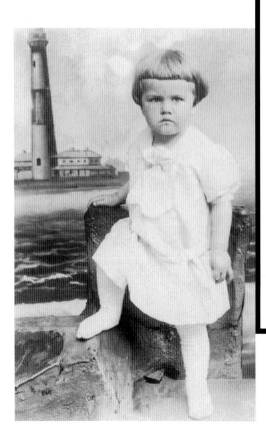

c.1924-1926

Baby Cut

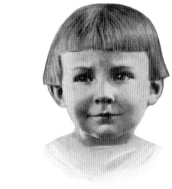

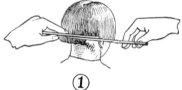

①

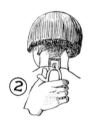

②

This style is worn by small children generally and little boys especially. It should be cut as follows:

FIRST:—Part the hair in the middle and brush smoothly all around. Start the hair line about the middle of the ear, or higher if desired, and cut a straight line all around the head as shown in figure (1).

SECOND:—To form the bangs brush the hair down on the forehead starting about three-quarters of an inch from the hair line. Cut the bangs at a point of equal distance between the eyebrows and the hair line, or higher if desired. Be sure to make a straight line from temple to temple.

Remove fuzzy hair from the neck with fine sharp clippers, as shown in figure (2).

When the cut is finished, it should look exactly like the central figure.

The time required to complete this cut, should not exceed fifteen (15) minutes.

The Tonsorial Artist, 1924

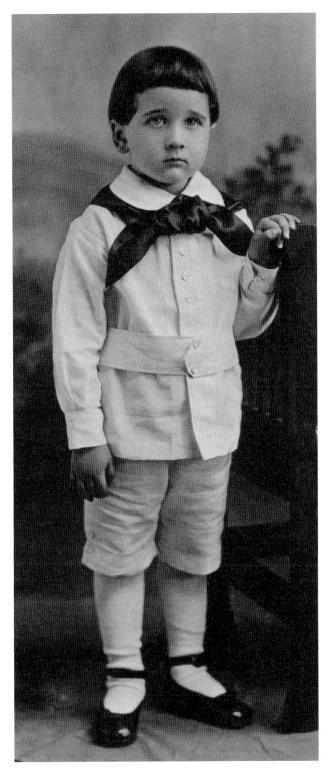

c.1919-1922

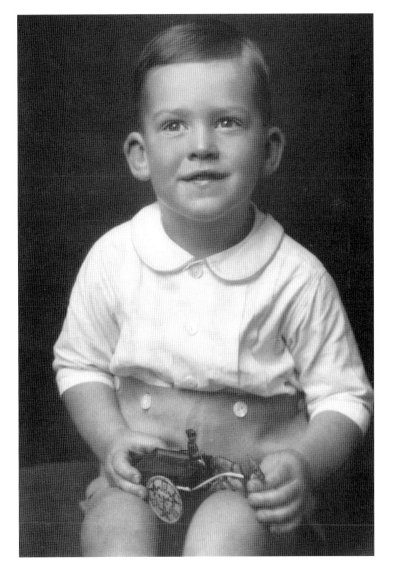

c.1929-1930

Chapter Five
Past Middle Age

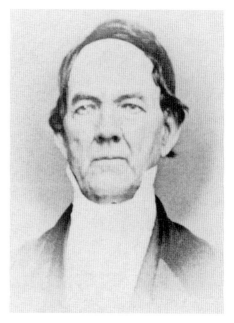

Introduction

Only on rare occasions did fashion magazines offer advice and information for the man or woman past middle age. Left to their own choices, aging Americans approached hairstyling from several directions. Some embraced comfort with little concern for the fashion rules of the young. Others attempted to stay abreast of the latest vogue, sometimes to the point of silliness. A few clung steadfastly to their own youth, becoming anachronisms of style and the butt of humor. Regardless of the choice, however, fashion was always more difficult for the older lady than for the older gentleman.

A photograph taken about 1864 in Baltimore reflects the hair and clothing of the mid 1850s on an elderly gentleman reluctant to change.

Ladies

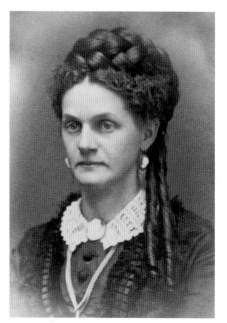

Many older women adopted the plain, practical bun, pulling their hair back with or without a part, depending on the preference of the day. From the 1830s through the early 1850s, lace head coverings were practically a requirement for the elderly lady. By the 1860s a headdress of narrow ribbons was favored.

Elaborate ladies' coiffures of the 1870s were seldom attempted with the thinning tresses of the elderly, while those of middle age found no difficulty in adapting variations of the popular styles to dressy occasions. Braids and curls were worn, along with decorative combs and modest adornments. The variety of the 1880s and its introduction of the pulled back twist brought relief to those no longer young enough to endure hours of fuss and frills. Hair now could be as simple or elaborate as one wished, and the older woman found she was no longer doomed to the ranks of the unfashionable.

Exaggerated coiffures of the 1870s were exceptionally silly on women of middle age or beyond.

The era of the Gibson Girl that began in the 1890s was both good and bad for the aging. The ease of the pompadour in its most basic form was a welcome change for the woman who had spent her youth struggling with the curling iron. But the amount of hair needed to achieve the lush new styles was a definite problem. The solution for the mature woman lay in modification—a look less full, and frequently more curly as the permanent wave became an accepted feminine convenience.

By World War I the wisdom of age had decreed that the shortest distance to true comfort was the simplest line. There were, after all, more interesting things to concern oneself with. The modern attitude for the lady of advancing years could now be summed up in the words scrawled at the bottom of a souvenir photograph of aging beauties vacationing in Santa Catalina—"We feel better than we look!"

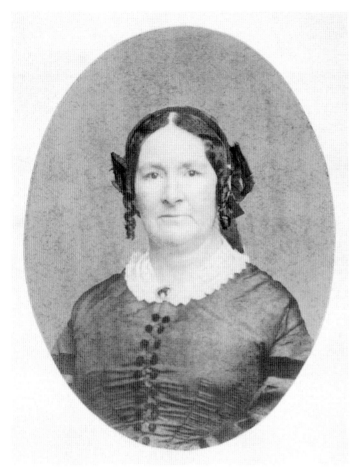

c.1858-1860

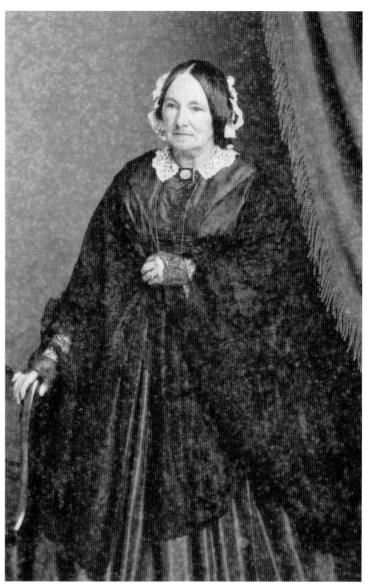

New York City, c.1860-1864

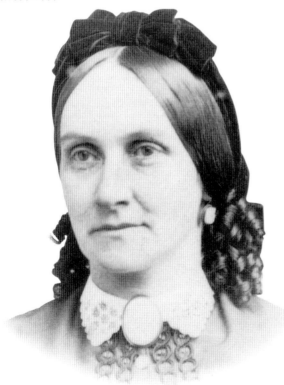

Philadelphia, Pa., c.1865-1867

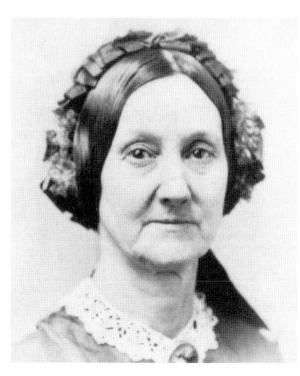

Baltimore, Md., c.1865-1867

169

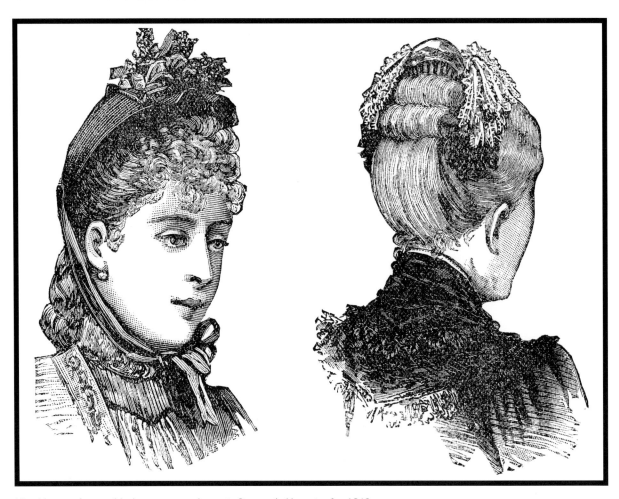

Headdresses for an elderly woman as shown in *Peterson's Magazine* for 1869.

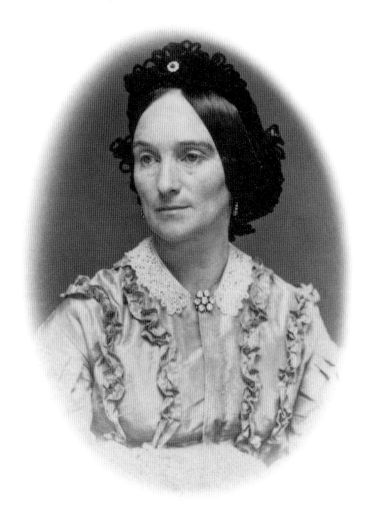

c.1865-1868

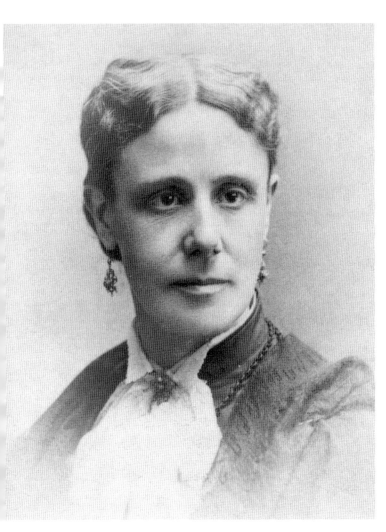

Trenton, N.J., c.1866-1868

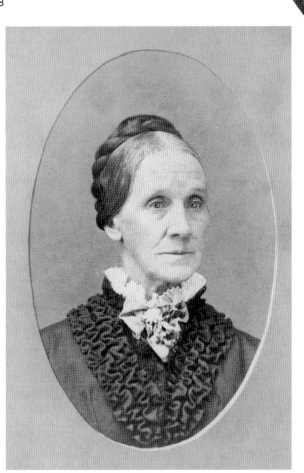

San Francisco, Calif.,
c.1872-1874

Somerville, N.J., c.1870-1874

171

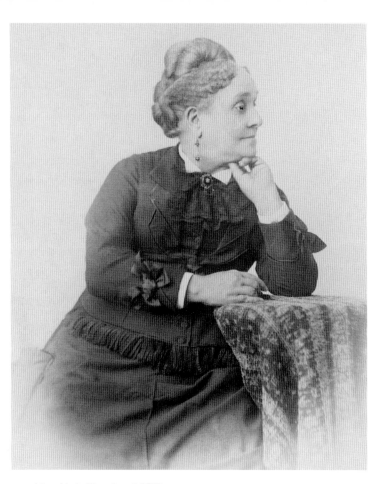

New York City, dated 1878

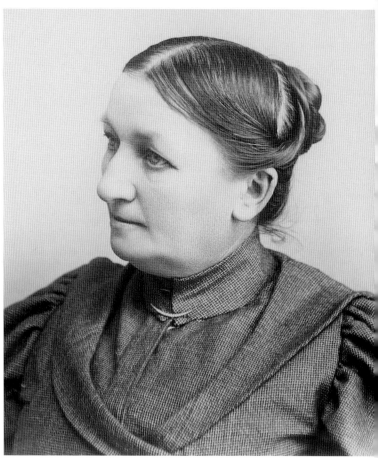

Dated 1878

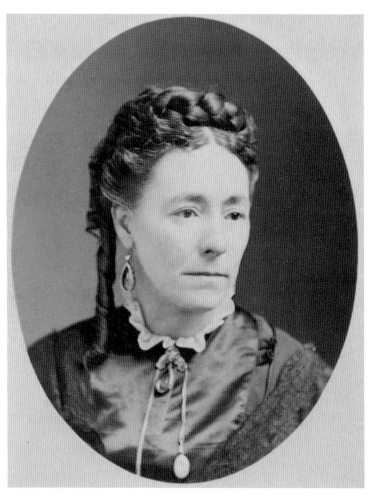

Carthage, N.Y., c.1871-1874

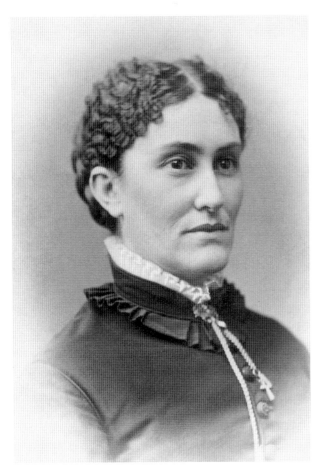

Mitford, Mass., c.1880-1883

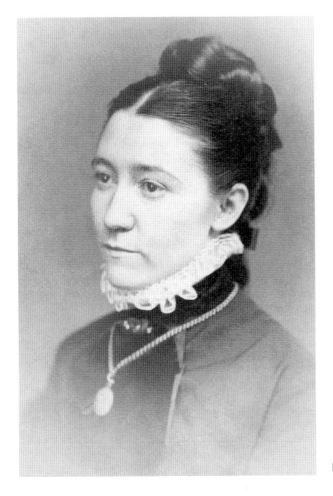

Indiana, Pa. c.1880-1883

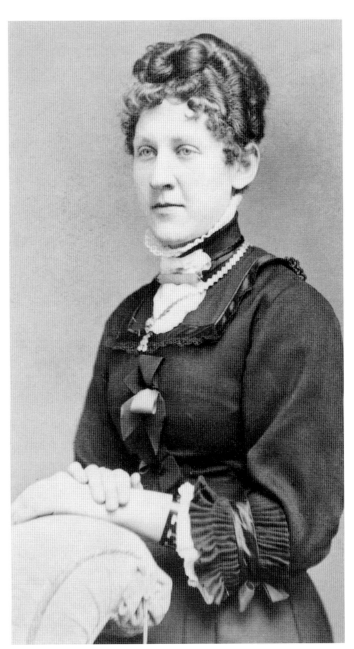

Jerseyville, Ill., c. 1883-1885

173

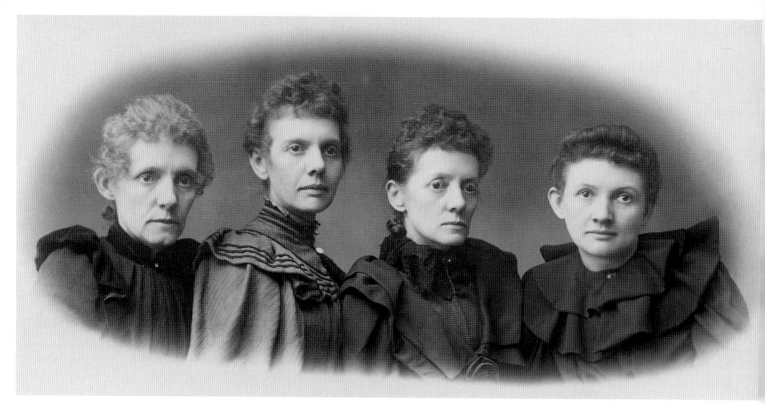

Greensburg, Pa., c.1896-1900

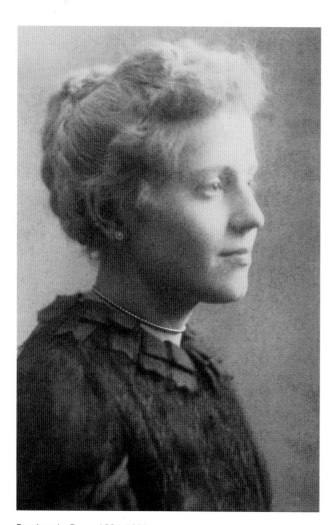

Pittsburgh, Pa., c.1896-1900

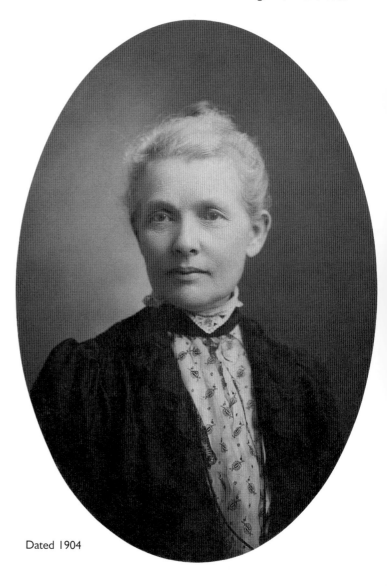

Dated 1904

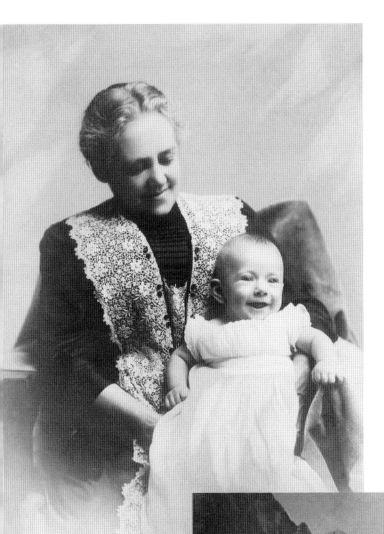

c.1910-1912

c.1910-1913

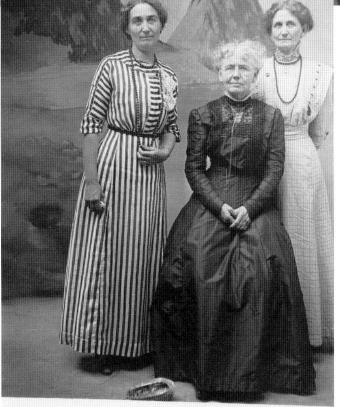

We feel better than we look.

Santa Catalina, c.1910-1913
"We feel better than we look."

175

Gentlemen

All but the most eccentric of older men accepted the fashions of the time, although more than a few wore them for too long. Even the stylish beards, sideburns and mustaches of the 1860s were adopted when seen on such notable figures as Robert E. Lee and Ulysses S. Grant.

From the 1880s to World War I, what a man wore on his head was less the fashion focus than what he wore on his face. The same held true for the older American. The very mature man of the 1880s often adopted a beard. In the 1890s his choice was more than likely to be a mustache. By the turn of the century only college professors, doctors, scientists, and the like affected beards. The mustache too was on its way out as the male world both old and young turned clean-shaven and sleekly coiffed to suit the modern era. Many found it was easier to retain at least the appearance of youth with the new, more natural looking hair dyes found so plentifully on the market. Age, it seemed, had become a matter of personal attitude, and a man was only as old as he felt.

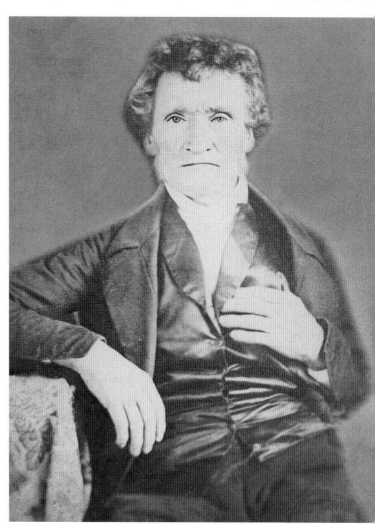

A suit worn far too long and a hairstyle suitable for a younger man date this image anywhere from the mid-1850s to the early 1860s.

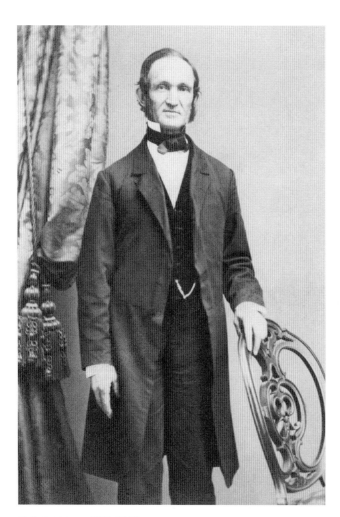

Philadelphia, c.1862-1863

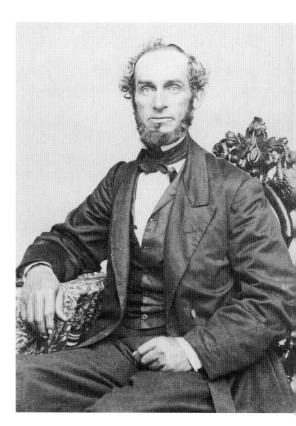

Syracuse, N.Y., dated 1867

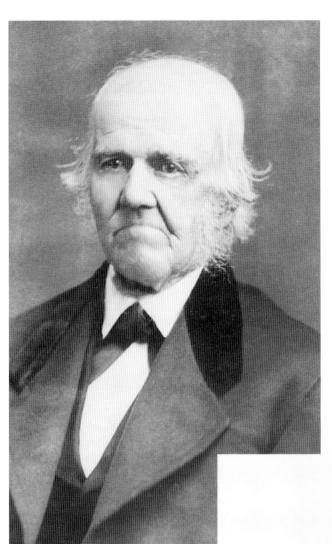

Mansfield, Ohio c.1876-1877

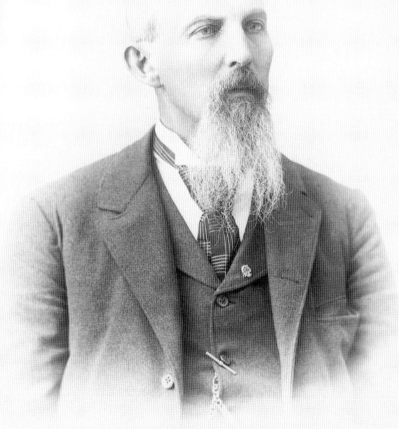

Racine, Wis., c.1878-1880

Pittsburgh, Pa., c.1880-1882

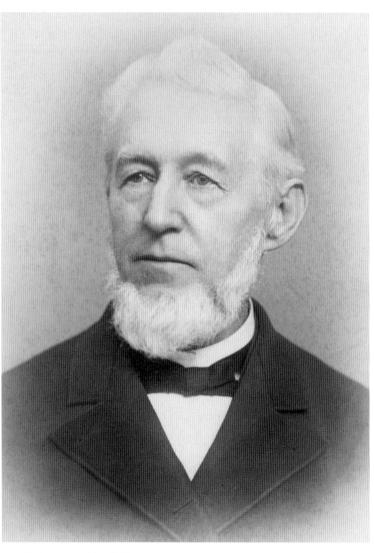

York, Pa., c.1884-1887

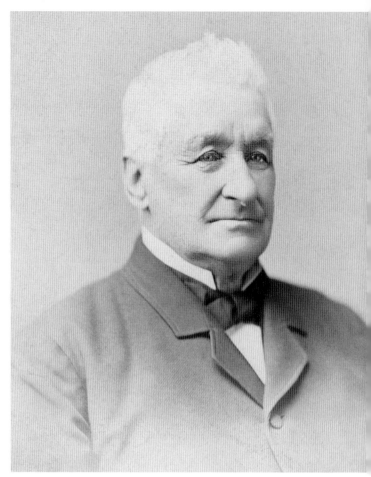

Hudson, N.Y., c.1883-1886

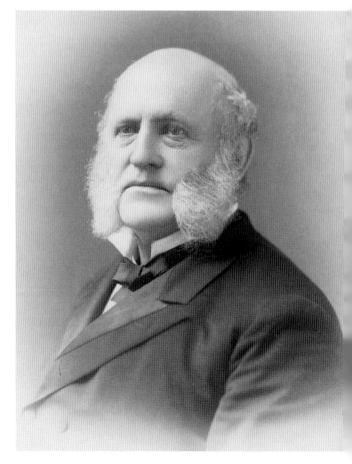

New York City, c.1886-1888

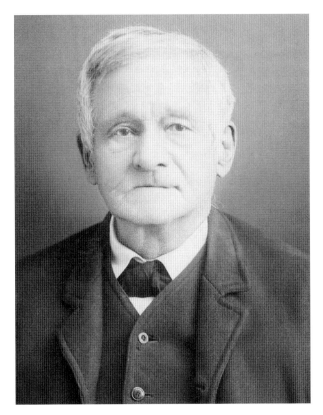

Canisteo, N.Y., c.1894-1898

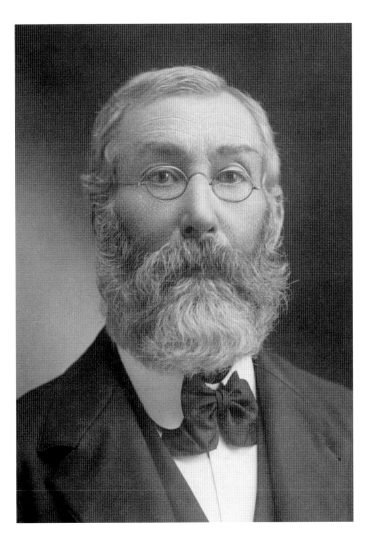

Zelienople, Pa., c.1912-1913

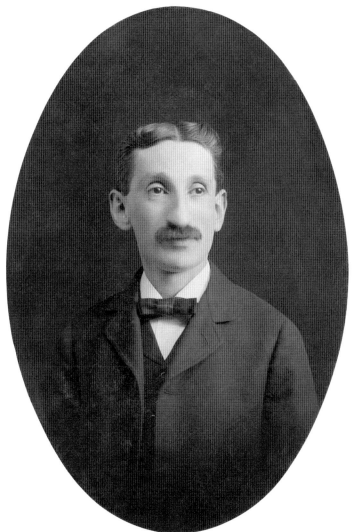

Pittsburgh, Pa., c. 1902-1910

179

Chapter Six
A Fine Head of Hair

"Hair left to take care of itself will revenge itself by making its possessor either common looking or a monster of ugliness," exotic beauty Lola Montez said in 1890. Possessing a fine head of hair was certainly a recognized goal for both men and women. It was women, however, who had the most arduous task. Even the simple act of brushing was made complex and demanding.

"Brush not one minute, but ten—not once a day, but two, three, or four times a day," Miss Montez advised. Two brushes were considered indispensable for the toilet; one for brushing, the other to smooth and polish. Two combs were also needed; a coarse toothed comb to loosen knots, and a fine toothed one to remove dust and the sweet scented orris powder many Victorian women sprinkled onto their scalp. One hundred brush strokes at the end of each day were believed necessary to keep the hair healthy and to provide a daily cleansing.

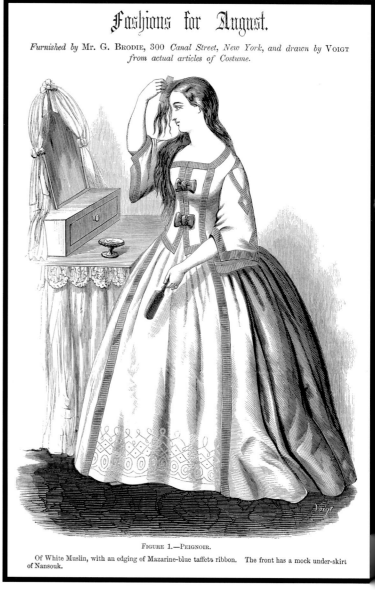

Fashions for August.

Furnished by Mr. G. Brodie, 300 Canal Street, New York, and drawn by Voigt from actual articles of Costume.

FIGURE 1.—PEIGNOIR.

Of White Muslin, with an edging of Mazarine-blue taffeta ribbon. The front has a mock under-skirt of Nansouk.

Harper's Monthly, 1861

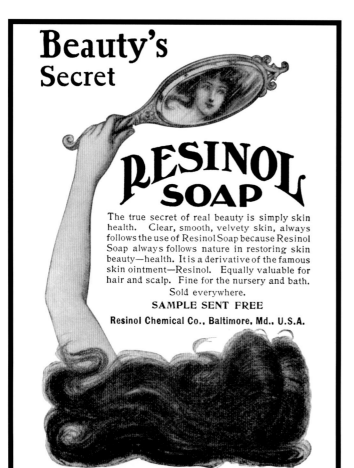

Beauty's Secret

RESINOL SOAP

The true secret of real beauty is simply skin health. Clear, smooth, velvety skin, always follows the use of Resinol Soap because Resinol Soap always follows nature in restoring skin beauty—health. It is a derivative of the famous skin ointment—Resinol. Equally valuable for hair and scalp. Fine for the nursery and bath.

Sold everywhere.

SAMPLE SENT FREE

Resinol Chemical Co., Baltimore, Md., U.S.A.

From *The Cosmopolitan*, 1903

Clean hair was not the priority in the past that it is today. For some, a monthly shampooing was considered more than adequate. "Shampooing is a great detriment to the beauty of the hair," one source warned. "Wash the scalp, but not the hair," another instructed, explaining how to sponge the roots with soapy water. Twice monthly washings were the norm despite such advice, and in warm weather the scalp was sponged frequently with an aromatic wash. Alcohol or ammonia, light oil, egg yolk, and fine soap dissolved in rainwater with a drop or two of perfume were common ingredients of such washes. Shampoos too could be homemade, though most women of the late Victorian period used either commercial cleansers or one of the popular bar soaps.

Once the hair was clean, something must be done with it. "Disheveled locks are rarely in fashion," an 1870 household book gravely reminded its feminine readers. But arranging the hair in the latest mode wasn't easy. Rippling waves could be produced by braiding the hair overnight. Curling or pressing tongs and crimping irons were a fast and effective aid, but their overuse was damaging. Putting sections up with strips of cloth at bedtime created curls that went limp again in short order. Even a wrapping of curling papers was ineffective without some sort of setting lotion.

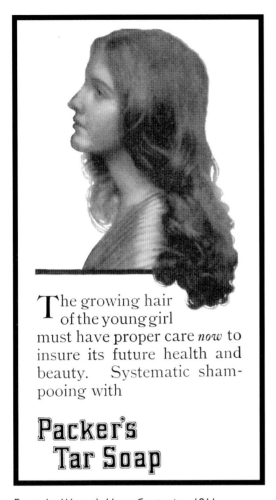

The growing hair of the young girl must have proper care *now* to insure its future health and beauty. Systematic shampooing with

Packer's Tar Soap

From the *Woman's Home Companion*, 1911

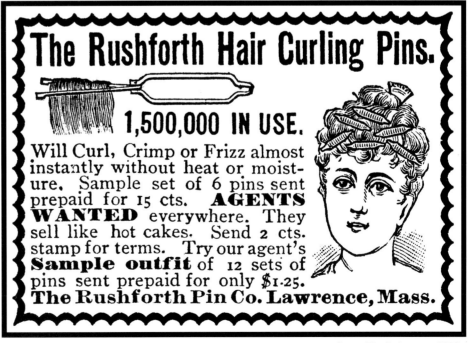

The Rushforth Hair Curling Pins.

1,500,000 IN USE.

Will Curl, Crimp or Frizz almost instantly without heat or moisture. Sample set of 6 pins sent prepaid for 15 cts. **AGENTS WANTED** everywhere. They sell like hot cakes. Send 2 cts. stamp for terms. Try our agent's **Sample outfit** of 12 sets of pins sent prepaid for only $1.25. **The Rushforth Pin Co. Lawrence, Mass.**

From *The Delineator*, 1895

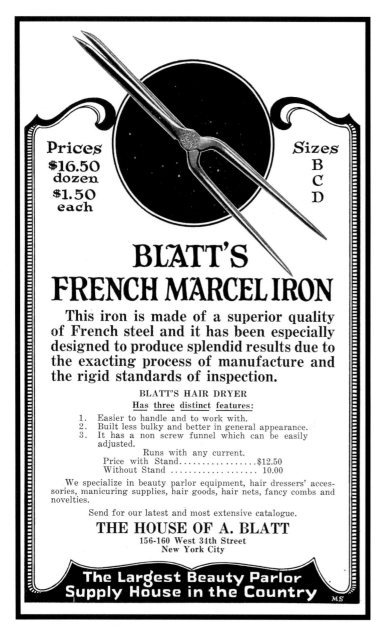

Above and right:
Curling and waving the modern way—from
The Tonsorial Artist, 1924.

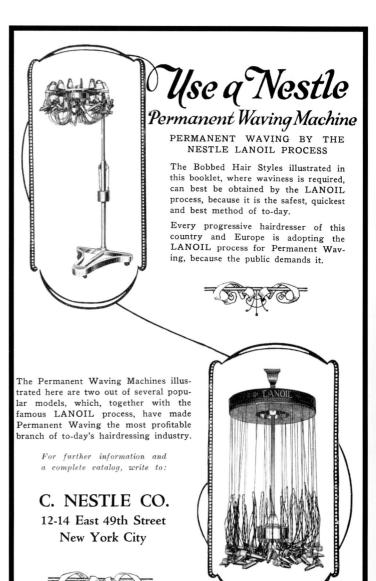

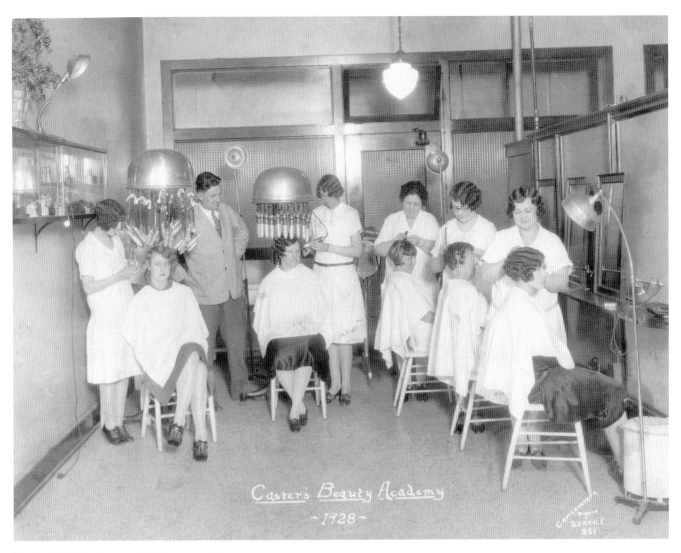

Modern Hairdressing at a 1928 beauty academy.

Many home recipes for setting lotions were based on water in which quince seeds had been boiled; others named gum arabic as a prime ingredient. Commercially these were called *fixateurs* or bandolines. To give the hair smoothness and sheen, a grease-based pomade or pomatum was worked in. Although a multitude of commercial products were available, many preferred the old tried and true recipes. One 1888 home guide called for the marrow of a beef shank to be melted in a double boiler, then strained and scented with attar of roses. An 1891 book insisted that bear's grease was as pleasant a pomatum as anything, but recommended rubbing the hair well with flannel before touching it to the pillow at night. Those who disliked the oiliness of pomades bought hair tonics such as Florida Water or Pinaud's, which promised not only glossy hair but a miracle or two as well.

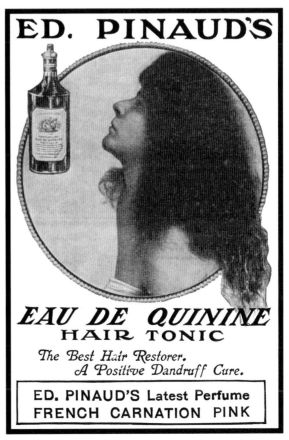

1901 magazine advertisement

Selling miracles was a lucrative pursuit during the Victorian and Edwardian eras, and barbers and druggists filled their shelves with colorful bottles of liquid promises. The man or woman with graying hair might use a homemade rinse from walnut husks. The bottle of commercial hair dye was likely to have been made from walnut husks as well—but it also promised youth in glowing terms. Many products claimed to actually restore the hair's original color and reinvigorate its growth.

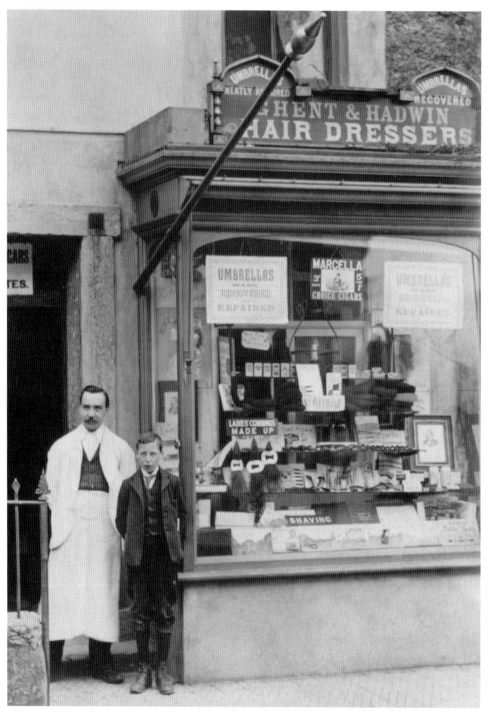

A hairdresser's window filled with hair care products, accessories, and miracle treatments of the early 1900s.

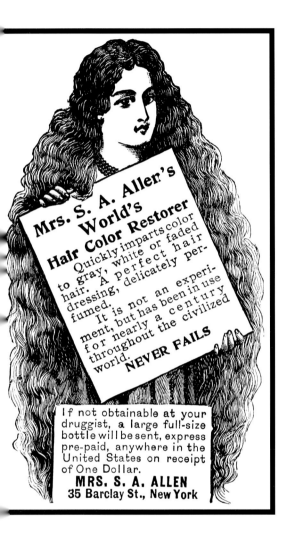

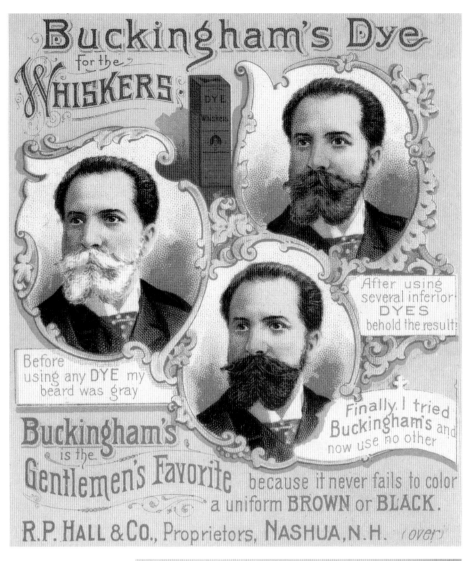

It was said that Caesar wore a laurel wreath to hide his baldness. Victorian men turned to wigs…not always with great success. They also searched for the elusive cure that would return to them what time and nature had stolen away. Hundreds of treatments were proposed over the years ranging from massage with a raw onion, to shaving the head for a rebuilding of strength. Those with faith in the technology of the modern age sent galvanic currents across the scalp or donned a lethal looking "vacuum" helmet guaranteed to stimulate hair growth.

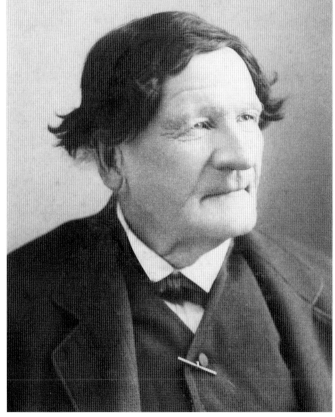

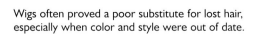
Wigs often proved a poor substitute for lost hair, especially when color and style were out of date.

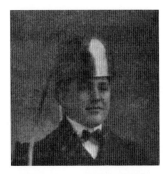
McClure's Magazine, 1903.

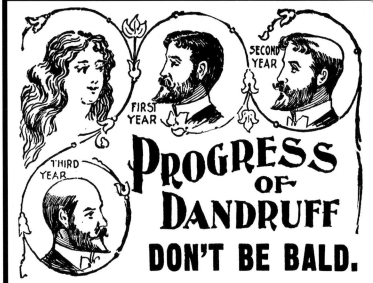
The Ladies' World, 1900
Dandruff was believed another cause of baldness.

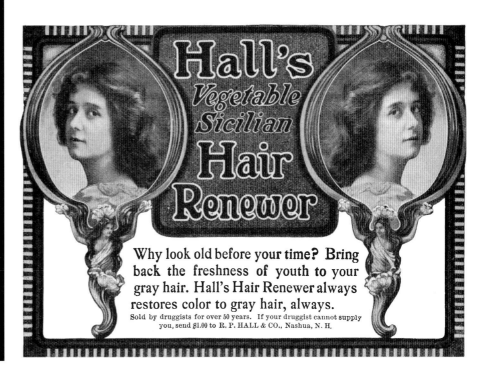

Marvelous Growth of Hair.

A Famous Doctor-Chemist Has Discovered a Compound That Grows Hair on a Bald Head in a Single Night.

The Discoverer Sends Free Trial Packages to All Who Write

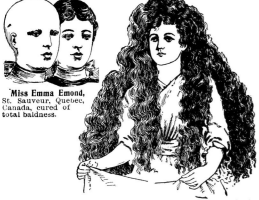

Miss Emma Emond,
St. Sauveur, Quebec,
Canada, cured of
total baldness.

MISS HISLOP of New Zealand and her marvelous growth of hair.

After half a century spent in the laboratory, crowned with high honors for his many world-famous discoveries, the celebrated physician-chemist at the head of the great Altenheim Medical Dispensary, 4857 Butterfield Bldg., Cincinnati, Ohio, has just made the startling announcement that he has produced a compound that grows hair on any bald head. The doctor makes the claim that after experiments, taking years to complete, he has at last reached the goal of his ambition. To the doctor all heads are alike. There are none which cannot be cured by this remarkable remedy. The record of the cures already made is truly marvelous and were it not for the high standing of the great physician and the convincing testimony of thousands of citizens all over the country it would seem too miraculous to be true. There can be no doubt of the doctor's earnestness in making his claims nor can his cures be disputed. He does not ask any man, woman or child to take his or anyone else's word for it but he stands ready and willing to send free trial packages of this great hair restorative to any one who writes to him for it, enclosing a 2 cent stamp to prepay postage. In a single night it has started hair to growing on heads bald for years. It has stopped failing hair in one hour. It never fails no matter what the condition, age or sex. Old men and young men, women and children all have profited by the free use of this great new discovery. Write to-day if you are bald, if your hair is falling out or if your hair, eyebrows or eyelashes are thin or short and in a short time you will be entirely restored.

This whole page:
Magazine advertisements and trade cards of the 1890's to 1903.

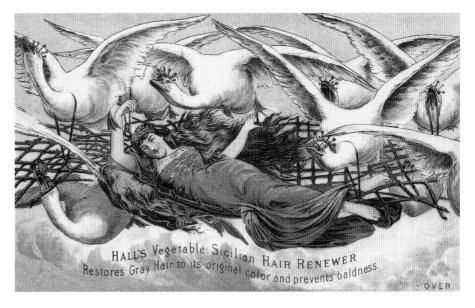

The more luxuriant the hair pictured in the advertisement, the more believable its claims. Possibly the most successful purveyors of hair products were the Seven Sutherland Sisters, each with floor length tresses. With their manager in tow, the Seven Sutherlands took to stages across the country in an elaborate publicity campaign that even modern advertisers would admire.

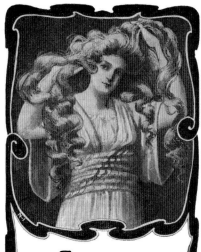

Seven Sutherland Sisters

HAIR GROWER and SCALP CLEANER

WILL not grow hair on a billiard ball; but where there exists a particle of life in a hair root, they will surely bring forth a strong, healthy hair. For nearly a quarter of a century they have been performing this noble work with increasing success.

The **Scalp Cleaner** makes a delightful creamy, cleansing, purifying lather, which is far superior and quite as economical as good soap.

The **Hair Grower** is an ideal tonic. It destroys microbes and completely eradicates dandruff. It restores the decaying hair roots, stops hair falling out, and keeps it healthful, soft and lustrous.

The only hair preparation that can be found in nearly every drug and department store in the United States.

Over 28,000 dealers sell them. Why? Permit us to again say :

It's the Hair-not the Hat
That makes a woman attractive

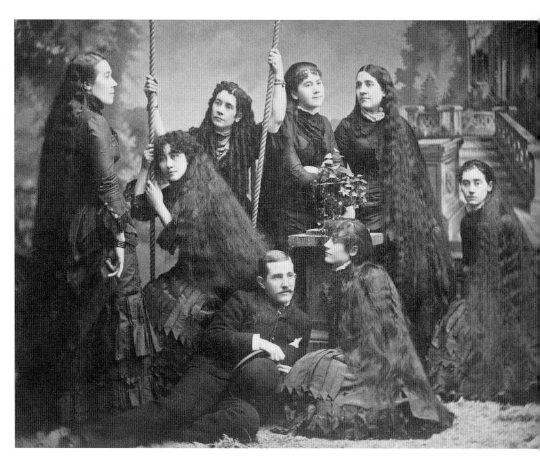

The Seven Sutherland Sisters and their manager.

Raised on superstition and old wives' tales, our ancestors were extremely gullible. They believed that long hair caused headaches, weakened the eyesight, and sapped the strength during illness—and surviving photographs of women and children with cropped heads attest to the cure. They also believed in a direct connection between the hair and the brain. "Numerous instances are on record in which disorders of a dangerous character have been removed by simply cutting the hair," *Godey's Lady's Book* asserted in 1867, adding that history also provided testimony concerning hair turned white overnight by traumatic shock.

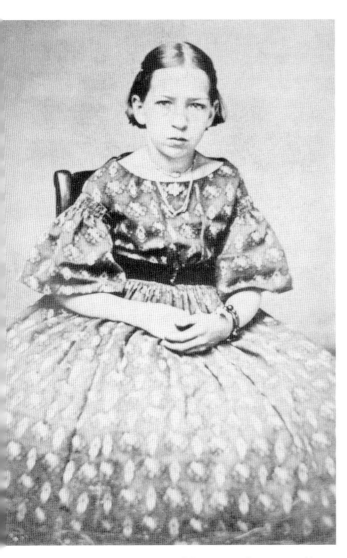

A treatment for certain types of illness was often cropped hair.

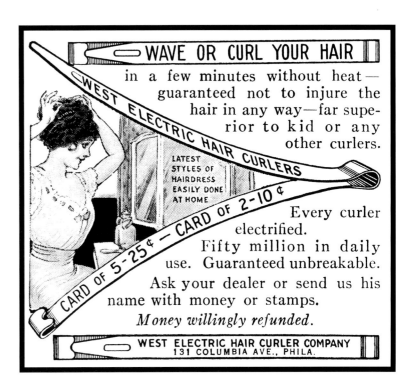

Above and below:
The gullible believed that electricity could impart near-magical properties.

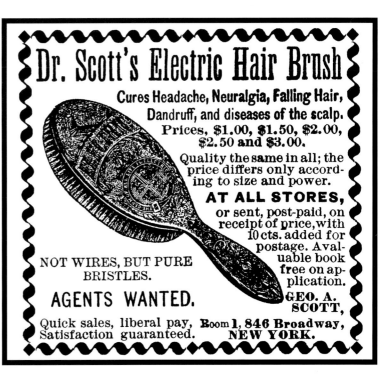

Many devoutly believed that the condition and color of the hair revealed the disposition of its wearer. Redheaded persons were quick of temper and unstable. Auburn or light brown hair indicated intelligence, industry, and a tender nature. Blondes were sensitive and delicate of constitution, although bleached hair was always equated with immorality. "Frizzly" hair warned of an adventurous, changeable character and fickle affections. Strong, coarse hair went with a coarse nature, while fine, glossy tresses accompanied refinement and morality. Lank, limp hair warned of "pusillanimity and cowardice."

It's no wonder then that people bought combs that promised to tint the hair, and "electric" hairbrushes and curlers that had never been touched with voltage. Electricity did finally produce the miracle of permanently waved and curled hair for the woman of the 1920s who bravely subjected herself to the tentacles of the beauty parlor machine in exchange for months of curler free style. The home permanent did nearly as well, though it might take eight messy hours or more to complete.

"The greatest ornament to the 'human form divine' is, unquestionably, a fine, luxuriant, healthy growth of hair," Godey's Lady's Book wrote in 1867. "It is to beauty of woman the chief auxiliary, and to manhood the warrant of strength and dignity." Throughout history, the head has been scorched, doused and tortured in endless ways—all in the name of vanity—and to keep every hair in place.

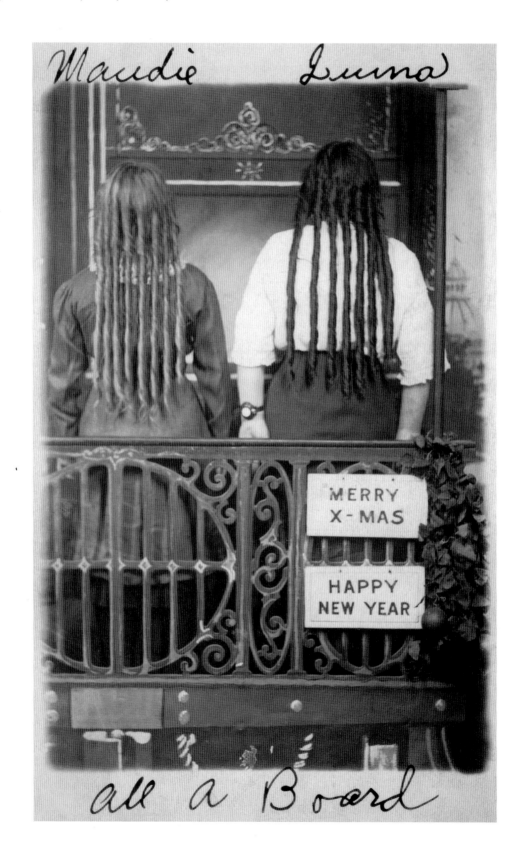

Bibliography

Blum, Stella, ed. *Fashions and Costumes from Godey's Lady's Book*. New York: Dover Publications, Inc., 1985.

Bouchot, Henri. "A Century of Fashions," *The Cosmopolitan*, July 1895.

Brinton, D. G., and George H. Naphys. *The Laws Of Health In Relation To The Human Form*. Springfield, Massachusetts: W. J. Holland, 1869.

Burton, Helen M. "Then and Now," *Peterson's Magazine*, October 1889.

"Chitchat on Fashions for July," *Godey's Lady's Book And Magazine*, July 1873.

"Curious And Useful Information," *American Homes*, January 1874.

Decorum: A Practical Treatise On Etiquette And Dress. Detroit: F. B. Dickerson & Co., 1879.

Editor's Drawer, *Harper's New Monthly Magazine*, September 1854.

Editor's Drawer, *Harper's New Monthly Magazine*, February 1858.

Editor's Table, *Peterson's Magazine*, February 1869.

Editor's Table, *Peterson's Magazine*, April 1869.

Editor's Table, *Peterson's Magazine*, August 1869.

Editor's Table, *Peterson's Magazine*, December 1869.

"False Hair," *Appleton's Journal*, 19 March 1870.

"A Few Words About Beards," *The Metropolitan*, April 1872.

Gernsheim, Alison. *Victorian and Edwardian Fashion: A Photographic Survey*. New York: Dover Publications, Inc., 1981.

"Good Taste and Bad Taste in Dressing the Hair," *The Ladies' Home Journal*, November 1908.

"Hair-Dressing," *Harper's Bazar*, 7 July 1889.

"Hair-Dressing And Neck Wear," *Harper's Bazar*, 2 March 1891.

Home And Society, *Scribner's Monthly*, September 1873.

Home And Society, *Scribner's Monthly*, September 1873.

Hoyt, Harlowe Randall. *Town Hall Tonight*. New Jersey: Prentice-Hall, Inc., 1955.

Kunciov, Robert, ed. *Mr. Godey's Ladies*. New York: Bonanza Books, 1971.

"Ladies' Head Gear," *Ballou's Dollar Monthly Magazine*, February 1863.

McClellan, Elizabeth. *Historic Dress In America 1607-1870*, 2 vols. New York and London: Benjamin Blom, Inc., 1904.

MAH' Studios. *The Tonsorial Artist: A Text-Book For Barbers And Hairdressers*, vol.1, 1st ed., New York: MAH' Studios, 1924.

Mallon, Isabel A. "Some Suggestions About The Hair," *The Ladies' Home Journal*, July 1892.

Melendy, Mary Ries. *Vivalore*. (n. p.): W. R. Vansant, 1904.

Mertin, Dr. Rudolph. "Hair Dyeing and Bleaching," *Beauty*, November 1922.

Miscellany, *Appleton's Journal*, 5 February 1870.

Morgan, Hal and Andreas Brown. *Prairie Fires And Paper Moons: The American Photographic Postcard: 1900-1920*. Boston: David R. Godine, 1981.

Moorshead, Halvor, ed., *Dating Old Photographs 1840-1929*. Toronto, Canada: Moorhead Magazines Ltd., 2000.

Notes And Queries, *The Dining Room Magazine*, May 1877.

"Now Open," *The Apollo News Record*, 26 June 1914.

Palmer, Corliss. "The Beauty Box," *Beauty*, November 1922.

Powel, Sarah. "Some French Fashions Of Other Days," *Peterson's Magazine*, September 1889.

"Quiptic Writings," *Men's Wear: 75 Years of Fashion*, 25 June 1965.

Ross, Ishbel. *Crusades And Crinolines*. New York: Harper and Row, 1963.

Schroeder, Joseph J., Jr. *The Wonderful World Of Ladies' Fashions 1850-1920*. Northfield, Illinois: Digest Books, Inc., 1971.

"Taste In Hair-Dressing," *The Dining Room Magazine*," December 1877.

Tomes, Robert. "Women's Form," *Harper's Monthly*, 1868.

Thorpe, Rose Hartwick. *As Others See Us*. Detroit: F. B. Dickerson Co., 1890.

VanAuken, Ida Cleve. "The New Ways to Fix Your Hair," *The Ladies' Home Journal*, February 1913.

Varieties, *Appleton's Journal*, 19 March 1870.

Varieties, *Family Herald*, November 1902.

Varney, Ruth. "Red Hair In All Ages," *Beauty*, November 1922.

Ward, Mrs. H. O. *Sensible Etiquette Of The Best Society: Customs, Manners, Morals, and Home Culture*. Philadelphia: Porter and Coates, 1878.

Wells, Richard A. *Manners, Culture and Dress of the Best American Society*. Springfield, Massachusetts: King, Richardson and Co., 1891.

"What to Wear," *Cassell's Family Magazine*, February 1888.

White, Annie Randall. *Twentieth Century Etiquette: An Up-To-Date Book For Polite Society*. n. p., 1900.

Young, John H. *Our Deportment: On the Manners, Conduct And Dress Of The Most Refined Society*. Detroit: E. B. Dickerson and Co., 1881.

General Fashion References

Beauty, November 1922.

Beautiful Womanhood, April 1923.

The Delineator, March 1895.

The Delineator, May 1895.

The Delineator, March 1911.

Frank Leslie's Ladies' Magazine And Gazette Of Fashion, January 1868.

Godey's Lady's Book, January-February 1841.

Godey's Lady's Book, bound, July—December 1850.

Godey's Lady's Book, bound, March—December 1867.

Godey's Lady's Book and Magazine, bound, July—December 1873.

Graham's Magazine, November 1841.

Harper's Bazar, 7 March 1868.

——. 5 February 1870.

——.17 February 1872.

——. 20 April 1872.

——. 20 December 1873.

——. 10 April 1880.

——. 15 May 1880.

——. 20 November 1880.

——. 5 March 1881.

——. 18 June 1881.

——. 9 July 1881.

——. 1 October 1881.

The Lady's Book, bound, May 1833—May 1834.

The Ladies' Home Journal, May 1891.

——. July 1892.

——. February 1895.

——. October 1898.

——. April 1899.

——. October 1901.

——. April 1915.

——. April 1916.

The Ladies' World, January 1894.

——. February 1894.

——. March 1894.

——. November 1894.

——. December 1899.

——. April 1900.

McCall's Magazine, June 1908.

——. August 1908.

——. November 1909.

——. August 1911.

——. January 1913.

——. August 1922.

Peterson's Magazine, bound, January—December 1869.

——. March 1870.

——. January 1889.

——. August 1889.

——. September 1889.

——. October 1889.

——. November 1889.

Woman's Home Companion, April 1902.

Woman's Home Companion, April 1906.

Woman's Home Companion, May 1911.